AF797257

A Kitchen You Love

Creating The Heart Of Your Home

Ann McKinley

AM-PM Publishing

AM-PM Publishing
116 Charles St.
Gordonsville VA 22942

First paperback printing September 2019

ISBN 978-0997119824

Contents

"Anyone can throw pretty cabinets against a wall and make it look good. Real success in a kitchen design is when you love it three years later *because* it functions so well."

-- Ann McKinley

For Paul,
Who is my ardent cheering section, leads by example, and allows me to be me.

Testimonials

"When the idea of creating a kitchen in our small church was first brought up, Ann jumped on it. Ann had the design skills and knowledge to see the project to completion. I was one of the volunteers who showed up regularly to help out and I have to say I learned a lot just working around her. Ann has supplied a wealth of knowledge on kitchen design in this book and I want to give her a shout out "Cool Beans!"

— Russell Jones
US Army Ret

"I bought a home that Ann designed. She has a creative flare for creating a highly functional space. There were several preparation areas conveniently located close to the sink and main appliances and the pantry with a bookcase was an unexpected delight. This book will prove invaluable whether you are designing your own kitchen or working with a consultant. It has all the information you need to design a kitchen you will love for years to come."

— Maria Callison

Author of *Among the Grackle*

Acknowledgements

First I must thank my husband Paul who has put up with my many questions about book writing and who is my go to person for computer help when I get in trouble.

I also want to thank my many customers who trusted me with their homes and their dreams..

Chapter 1
Lemonade

"...architecture is my delight, and putting up, and pulling down, one of my favorite amusements."
— Thomas Jefferson

This is a book on functionality

You won't see a lot of pretty pictures of cabinets, counters and appliances because functionality is often less obvious. Understanding how a kitchen functions requires reading between the lines to get to the true meaning. You have to dig past the surface fluff and see if there is any substance underneath. If your aim is to have a showcase kitchen and really don't ever intend to work in it, maybe this is not the book for you. There are a number of books out there with pretty pictures and a lot of fluff for ideas on style. Don't get me wrong, a highly functional kitchen should still look great. It is just that looks are not the target of this book. Frank Lloyd Wright's boss, Louis Sullivan stated "Form follows Function". Get the function down and then work on the 'form' (or looks) within the constraints of the function.

Well, "duh", you say "of course it has to be functional". But there is more to this than the basic refrigerator, stove, countertop, cabinets and don't forget the kitchen sink. All these components (plus some) are needed for a functional kitchen but they are also components of a dysfunctional kitchen.

Why write a book on functionality? It is so easy to get functionality wrong and it can make the difference between loving your new kitchen and wanting to remodel again just a few years later. Look at it this way, whether you are creating gourmet meals or just warming up leftovers, there needs to be an order, or flow to the process. How the space functions will allow you to proceed in a smooth manner. Yes, a person is likely to use their kitchen in different ways throughout the year. Sometimes it may be a party kitchen where friends gather to talk and munch on snacks. Other times it may be a place where the kids gather after school to work on homework while dinner is being prepared. There may be the occasional formal dinner where you want the mess of the kitchen closed off or there may be a caterer that will need to use the space. Then there are the big family gatherings where one person may be creating their specialty while another ices a cake and a third is at the pastry board cutting biscuits. The kitchen wears many hats and must easily handle each.

Think about the way you use your kitchen. There may be one predominant use with a couple of other activities thrown in. Would you actually use your kitchen differently if you had a nicer space? Maybe you would have more friends over and you would end up in the kitchen as mentioned above. Maybe you want to take a gourmet cooking classes but your kitchen is just too awkward to work in. This information is of prime importance to your designer and will be the start for your design.

What makes a dysfunctional kitchen

A dysfunctional kitchen may have one main flaw or just an accumulation of many small irritations. But any kitchen that makes you want to throw things across the room needs to be changed (this is the voice of experience).

One litmus test to determine functionality of the space is how easy the kitchen is to use. Are utensils stored where you use them, and are they readily accessible? Some examples of this would be potholders close to the oven, spatulas and stirring spoons close to the cooktop, spices and mixing bowls next to the prep area. Sometimes items need to be divided and stored in two locations for easy access. If there is a separate oven and cook top spaced more than a step apart, potholders may need to be stored in both areas.

A detail that is often overlooked is lighting; is it adequate? Well this one needs to be more than adequate. If the light is not where you need it, there can be dangerous consequences. Check out the chapter on electrical for more information.

What about traffic flow? Some kitchens really take the "heart of the home" literally and have 3 or 4 main arteries into the area. Other times there is an island that is immovably in the way between two main work areas. More on this in the chapter on traffic flow.

However the most frequent complaints are usually lack of storage and counter space. There are some good pointers covered in the chapter on cabinets about storage and there are some rules-of-thumb to use for counter space in the chapter on countertops.

Does any of this sound like your kitchen? You may have a few more problem areas to add to the list, but you get the point. Your new kitchen should overcome all these obstacles to being a functional kitchen. The following chapters will go into more detail on what to expect from a highly functional kitchen

Not sure if your kitchen is dysfunctional

So you don't know if you have a dysfunctional kitchen? Maybe you have not moved as many times as I have and experienced so many kitchens to be able to make a distinction, but if you have ever lived in an apartment you have probably experienced a dysfunctional kitchen.

I have lived in 15 homes so far in my life. This includes apartments, rental duplexes, mobile home, RV, houses I have bought and one I actually built. I remodeled 3 of the kitchens, so I've worked in a total of 18 kitchens. From the experience with these 18 kitchens, I have familiarity with all kinds of dysfunction from inadequate plugs and counter space to wall cabinets so low my mixer would not fit under it. I have seen and lived most of it but I imagine there are other inadequacies I have not experienced but maybe you have. As you read through the chapters I will expand on some of the problems I have personally encountered with kitchens and how they can be overcome.

Let's look at a typical apartment kitchen as an example of a dysfunctional kitchen. It is usually what is called a "galley" kitchen. This means there are cabinets on two facing sides. The sink is usually on one side and the range and refrigerator are on the other. Maybe there is a small pantry at the end of the sink cabinet run. The main dysfunction of this type of kitchen is usable countertop

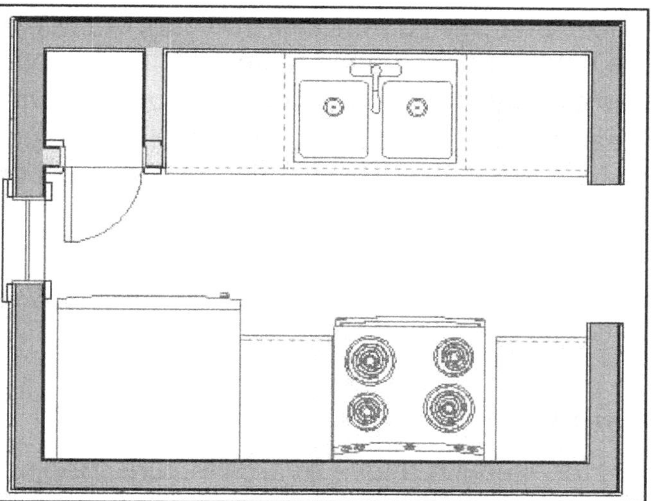

Typical Apartment Kitchen

and limited cabinet space. The countertop is usually 2 feet on one side of the sink which houses the dishwasher and 1 – 2 feet on the other side of the sink along with a 2 foot wide pantry. The facing wall has a standard range and refrigerator which allows for 1 1/2 foot counter on each side of the range. As you will find out in the countertop chapter, a 2 foot stretch is not long enough for a prep area. The cabinets themselves are usually very small with limited storage area. The one saving grace about apartments such as these is that they do have a pantry however small and inadequate.

Ok, Ok, I hear you. You are not living in an apartment but a home you own which is why you are considering remodeling. But you want to know if you can just paint what you have and maybe put in a new countertop and appliances and call it a remodel. You can, but will that get you the usable space you really need? The functionality remains exactly the same. Stop and consider what you have read so far. Does your kitchen really function well? Is it easy to maneuver in? Can you easily reach all your supplies? Is pie really easy to make in this space? Keep reading and you may discover the specific irritations that are causing you to dislike your kitchen and the remedies to create a kitchen you love.

Who am I

I started life with a love of architecture. Beginning at the age of 4, I would draw houses in my free time. I drew houses on paper taped together for my Barbie's to walk through, all the way to chalk houses on the driveway that *I* could walk through. The first section I read in the newspaper each Sunday was the housing section, even before reading the comics. I read books about designing and building your own house. I bought magazines of house designs and wore the covers off of them - many I still have, coverless. So when I graduated from High School I went to college and majored in - Food Science and Technology! Don't get me started on this but I did enjoy the major and learned a lot about food. But this major was not where I wanted to be so I went back to college and majored in – Mechanical Engineering! I don't know why someone never suggested architecture and you know what they say about hind sight. Well, broke and two degrees under my belt I had to start working. I bought my first house while working as an Aerospace Engineer for Kelly AFB in San Antonio Texas. I learned a lot about house maintenance then. I was doing so much that I had fellow male engineers drop by just to see what I was up to and I would get their muscle involved in helping me caulk the chimney or installing a new garbage disposal or putting in a garage door opener. I was bored and started working on a Masters in Human Factors Engineering, then I met my husband Paul (who helped me spread sand in my yard) and the fun really began.

While we were engaged, Paul took a job in Austin and put his home on the market. I thought I better get busy and sell my house after seeing how long it was taking Paul to sell his home. Well I listed mine 'For Sale by Owner' and the first day it came out in the paper it sold. We bought a duplex in Austin which allowed us to live rent free. When another duplex two houses down came on the market we jumped on it. Paul travelled a lot for business, so I performed a lot of the maintenance on these duplexes myself.

When I met Paul, he had a small plane and kept it in his backyard where he had a 'through-the-fence' use of a runway that ran behind the houses. Paul really wanted the same setup in Austin. There was an airport community in Austin but it was full so he decided Austin needed a new one. That was the start of Cross Country Estates, an airport community that we built near Georgetown Texas which is just north of Austin. We did much of the work ourselves. I personally never ran the grader and never got the hang of double clutching the dump truck but I did enjoy the backhoe and shredding the field by pulling the batwing mower behind the tractor which was very soothing. Soon after buying the 68 acres we brought in a small used mobile home to live in. This was a 2 bedroom, 2 bath, 924 square foot home. The kitchen would not meet the criteria I have now but for the moment it served well. One quirk I really enjoyed in that kitchen that I have not been able to repeat yet in a house was a gas cook top and electric oven.

At this time I was working for a small MEP firm in Austin. MEP stands for mechanical, electrical and plumbing. Some of the more memorable projects during this time were designing the plumbing for the restrooms of a baseball complex and designing the electrical system for the Barbara Jordan Elementary School. When the contractor reviewed the drawings I submitted for the school, he was amazed that I had actually listened to the request that were made and found a way to get them in the plan. I guess he was not used to getting what he wanted.

As the airport community took shape, I was able to design a house for my family which now numbered 3, and build it on one of the lots in the subdivision. This was the first kitchen I was able to design from scratch. I never took pictures of this kitchen because at the time I had no idea that I would be designing kitchens for others.

I also created a portfolio of house plans with attached hangers to get the ideas flowing with perspective lot purchasers. This did give many the idea of how to attach the hangar to the house they wanted.

We eventually moved farther up the highway to the small community of Morgan's Point Resort City (MPRC). Housing was cheap there and we bought a larger house than we previously had for a lot less, but then again, it needed a lot of work. I know that the color white is popular right now in 2016 but this house had been painted ALL white: walls, trim, ceiling all the same color, flat, stark, white. We even found the cans in the shop and they said 'white' not oyster, not antique just white. It was depressing. When we got some color on the walls I was feeling more hopeful. I will expand on this kitchen in the next several chapters. Let me just say the kitchen we inherited in this house was bad. It was the one I got so frustrated in I would throw things.

During our stay in MPRC I received my real estate license and started selling real estate. I enjoyed showing all the houses, but was always dismayed at the new homes with problem kitchens. I was told not to point out the potential problems because they were not 'materially substantial' and I did not want to plant doubts in the mind of a potential buyer, if they were true problems the buyer would notice. I had to bite my tongue.

Later we made the big move to Virginia where housing is a lot more expensive but we were able to find a MAJOR fixer-upper very cheap. As of this writing we are in the middle of bringing this house back to health. Hey, we now have running water! That's just to let you know how bad it was.

I have also taken a class in Net Zero Energy Houses. This is a very interesting and fast growing field.

Why am I interested in kitchen design

Housing is a passion of mine. As you can tell from my background I have always had an interest in housing. This interest has taken various forms through the years. Not only have we owned and lived in many homes but we have owned various rental properties. Our many acquisitions often required renovating to either bring the house back to health or just to get it into the right decade.

Often that renovation involved the kitchen and bathrooms. The most complicated rooms in a house are the kitchen, bathroom, and laundry as they require lots of plumbing, specific lighting and more complicated electrical than any of the other rooms. This is a challenge I am prepared for due to my experience with housing and my background in mechanical engineering and even the food science degree comes into play.

My experience in real estate has also been an education for me. Whenever I would go into a house, I would mentally critique the kitchen; paying attention to how it functioned as a work space and how it did not. The extra classes I have taken from Human Factors Engineering to Net Zero Energy Houses have also given me insights in how to make the most expensive room of the house function more comfortably for the occupants.

There is no reason to live with a dysfunctional kitchen. Improvements can be made.

What I hope you get out of this book

The design process is more than putting pretty cabinets against the wall. Yes that is part of it, but there is so much more to consider.

Each chapter will delve into a facet of design and how it is functionally important. Some techniques may be simple and inexpensive to implement but unfortunately bringing the best functionality to a space may get complicated which translates into money. There is only so much you can do to a space that resembles the above apartment kitchen without spending a lot of money. Sometimes the kitchen must be rearranged or walls may even need to be moved or removed. But keep your eye on the goal and soon you will have a kitchen you enjoy working in.

Remember there will always be problems

I don't want to sound negative but this is just a fact in the renovation construction field. Even in new constructions there will be problems. Just treat it like a challenging puzzle and don't take it personally. The carpenter may measure twice but still make the wrong cut, a sheet of expensive tiles are dropped and broken, a 2x4 may be warped beyond use; these things happen. This is why you always order 10% more materials than you think you will need. There's a reason the construction field is a major contributor to the landfill. Even when everyone is doing their job correctly, the cabinets may still come in with the wrong doors. Therefore also apply the 10% rule to time not just materials.

In rehabbing houses it got to where my husband and I would cringe whenever we opened a wall. We never knew what problem we would find. Maybe I should rephrase that – We never knew what challenge we would encounter.

Sometimes we would run into shoddy work from a previous owner or contractor (yes not all contractors do great work). One time we opened a wall to find 17 nails hand driven into a 2x4 – I figured someone was having a bad day. Another wall in an upstairs addition was not sitting on a sill plate but the 2x4 wall framing was nailed directly to the floor joist and ceiling rafters. We even developed a phrase for this type of discovery; we called it a "What were they thinking". On another house the previous owner had fixed a leak in a water line by skipping the

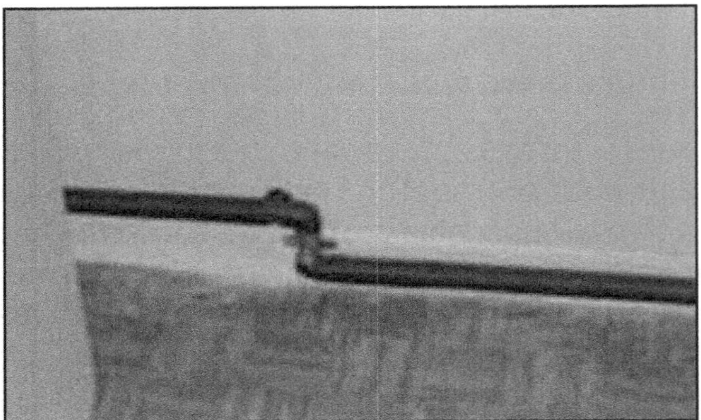

Exposed Plumbing

hassle of running the new piping in the wall and elected to bring the pipe outside the house, around the corner and back in to plumb the powder room downstairs. This was in Texas but we would still get freezing temperatures in the winter. As you can see in the picture, the pipe comes into the room and then divides to feed the toilet and the sink. Note the insulation on the interior piping shown while the exterior had none at all.

Even just recently while my husband was upstairs taking the walls down to the studs in a bathroom we were remodeling I heard him exclaim “Oh man!” I yelled up “What’s wrong”. He answered back “I just wish I could open one wall up and not have to rebuild it”. This particular wall was a load bearing wall that had studs that did

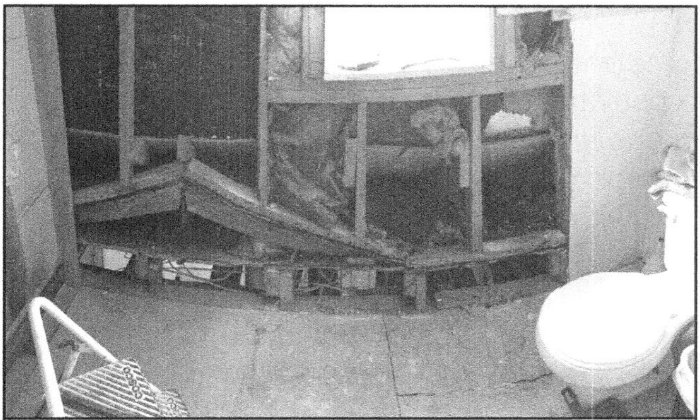

Faulty Framing

not go all the way from ceiling to floor! That was not the only problem with this wall, it was also out of plumb; leaning out at the top by 3 inches. 3 inches! I knew this was a problem from the beginning as there was a large glob of caulk in the corner to fill in where the square drywall did not touch.

Sometimes the problem is due to the age of the home. Codes are constantly changing and what was acceptable 40 years ago may not fly today. I just worked on a house that was built in the 80's but there were no GFI plugs in the kitchen!

Also insects may take a toll on the home. We opened the walls (meaning pulled the drywall off) in a kitchen remodel and discovered termite damage with live termites. What was strange about this was the 2x4s that looked the worst felt very solid but there were a couple 2x4s that looked perfect on the outside, but you could poke your finger through. The termites preferred the inner wood on those.

Sometimes there is a construction issue that makes it too costly to stay with your original design. I was working on one kitchen where we were trying to increase the storage space by replacing the existing 30 inch tall wall cabinets with 42 inch tall cabinets. The existing wall cabinets had a fur-down above them. (For those unfamiliar with the term, a fur-down or bulkhead is the boxed in filler between the top of the cabinets and the ceiling.) The fur-down had to be removed to allow the taller cabinets. In removing one fur-down we discovered the cast-iron soil pipe for the upstairs bathroom running through it. This meant a design change as moving the plumbing was too costly for this project. (You can do pretty much anything if you are willing to throw enough money at it). You have to remain flexible. Luckily we had not ordered the cabinets yet.

We were able to make lemonade out of the above challenge. While the plumber was on the job to re-plumb the sink, he noted that the cast iron drain pipe from the upstairs bathroom was starting to leak. So some problems may just be due to age, some things do wear out – even cast iron. It was lucky that he spotted the leaking. I couldn't imagine finishing this kitchen and then six months latter having bad smells and water stains in the ceiling! When you uncover a problem, fix it then!

The lemonade came on this particular kitchen when we reinstalled the soffit but extended them past the wall

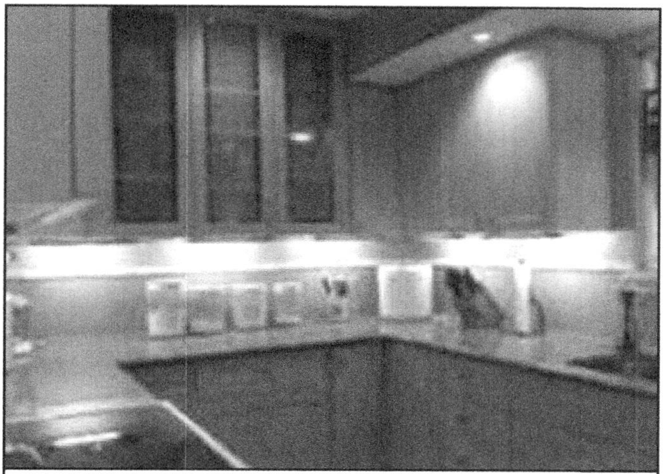

Extended Soffit & Can Light

cabinets and installed can lights in them. Since we were changing the kitchen from a galley style to a U shape we were able to put the taller 42" cabinets on the end wall and made it a feature by adding glass doors.

Go to https://akitchenyoulove.com/ch1 for a kitchen use checklist and to see the above pictures in color.

Chapter 2
In The Flow

"Simplicity, carried to an extreme, becomes elegance."
— Jon Franklin

Everything flows

There is a flow to life, there is a flow to music, and there is a flow to cooking. The family life flow just should not be down the middle of the kitchen. The kitchen may be the heart of the home but it doesn't have to be feeding a main artery. If all the daily traffic flows through the kitchen a detour is in order when the remodel is planned. The kitchen should not be treated as a hallway for safety reasons. There are hot pots being transported from the stove to the sink, there are pans on the range that are splattering hot grease, there are open dishwasher doors, there are hot dishes coming out of the oven and there are any number of other trip points and hazards to navigate around.

A kitchen only needs one or two entrances. I have seen homes with four to five doorways into the area. As of this writing I am working on a client's kitchen that has four entrances into the space. This is ridiculous. It would appear the kitchen was an afterthought of the builder who stuck it in a large hallway. There is an entrance to the dining room, an entrance to the family room, one to the utility room and another to a hall. What more could a person want? The challenge on this kitchen is I am not to move any walls or eliminate doorways. I have managed to come up with a design were I carved out an aisle for three of the doorways and now only have two real entrances into the kitchen. Luckily the client is not insisting on a doorway directly from the kitchen to the planned new outdoor deck. Even with two entrances into a kitchen I still like to see an alternate path around the kitchen.

Some kitchens have to act as a hallway; there is no other way to the utility room or the breakfast room. To change this would require a major renovation where walls are moved and maybe the kitchen moved to a different area. This can be done but much time and money would be involved. To move a kitchen would involve moving the plumbing. The supply lines may not be that hard to move if the home is on a crawlspace or basement foundation. And the drain lines might be manageable but there is another line called a vent that runs from the drain line inside the wall up through the roof. The vent is strategically placed in the drain line as-per-code and often not easily moved.

To move a kitchen will also involve moving the electrical. Though not as hard as the plumbing it may still involve running new wires from the electrical panel to accommodate additional lengths.

If the kitchen has to have two entryways and is the main path between areas, tuck the stove/oven/range into an out of the way area if at all possible. This is the most hazardous appliance in the kitchen. Pan handles stick out and can be knocked which could cause possible spills of very hot items. Oven doors may be left open while moving a dish to a table and cause a trip point and possible burns as someone tries to catch themself.

The refrigerator and the sink are often used by people coming from other parts of the house. Someone in the living room wants a cold drink so heads to the refrigerator. Make this appliance work in the flow so the occasional user does not have to trek to the middle or the heart of the kitchen for their drink. Stationing a second sink to a side area like a small minibar can also help keep traffic through the kitchen to a minimum.

So if at all possible plan for the kitchen to be a destination not a side attraction.

The work triangle.

The traditional work triangle is the imaginary triangle with its points at the sink, refrigerator and range. This is considered the main work area. The distance between these points are measured and added up, if it is more than 26 feet, too many steps have to be taken and the cook will be worn out by the end of the day. Keep it close and don't run a marathon trying to prepare a meal. The optimal distance for each leg of the triangle is between 4 and 9 feet. This is measured from the center of each appliance and sink.

I propose a different way of thinking about the work triangle. The above triangle works well for the cook who is always going back to the refrigerator, pulling one thing out at a time. But many cooks look at the recipe and go to the refrigerator pulling all the items at one time. In this case the refrigerator is treated as a cold pantry. This is the way I work. In this case, the work triangle shifts. The points now become the sink, the range and the preparation area. I worked in a kitchen once that had each leg of the sink, range and preparation triangle less than five feet and the refrigerator was off at the far end of the kitchen. This kitchen was a dream to work in. I could rinse my vegetables at the sink then turn 90 degrees and chop those vegetable in my preparation area then turn another 90 degrees and put them in the boiling water on the stove. I loved it. No wasted steps.

I have also seen a neighbor's new house and in looking at the kitchen (I always look at the kitchen) I realized there was no refrigerator. This is like looking under the hood of a car at a roomy engine compartment and realizing there is no battery or even a place for one. Where was the refrigerator? In the pantry of course! This pantry was not that close to the kitchen. It was about 10 feet away from the edge of the kitchen. I keep my freezer in the utility room but I am not ready to move the refrigerator out there with it.

I do advocate that the refrigerator be close to an entrance of the kitchen for two reasons. The refrigerator is often used by people other than the cook. Someone wants a cold drink and they go to the refrigerator. Someone wants a snack and they go to the refrigerator. Someone wants to make a sandwich and they go to the refrigerator. Some people prefer to install an additional small under counter refrigerator for others to use. This is good for drinks but does not satisfy the constantly hungry teenager who wants to stand in front of the open refrigerator looking for something to eat. Remember even these small refrigerator use a lot of electricity.

The second reason for stationing the refrigerator at the entrance of the kitchen is because it is large. That may sound like a strange reason. But the refrigerator blocks things. It blocks the flow of the kitchen work surfaces. If the refrigerator is between the sink and the range, the pot of hot water has to be pulled back and go around the refrigerator to be dumped in the sink. This can lead to spills in the floor or sloshed pots on the person carrying the pot. The refrigerator also blocks lights. I am big on adequate lighting in the kitchen but the elephant in the room cast shadows. Put the shadows on one side that is more out of the way.

Choose the work triangle that fits your mode of work in the kitchen. Considering the triangle in the kitchen layout can go a long way towards having an enjoyable cooking experience. It will make cooking less of a drudge.

Appliances have doors

These doors must be considered in the plan. Continuing the discussion on refrigerators above with the refrigerator blocking light and flow, the appliance also blocks aisles. This is the main drawback about putting it close to the entrance of a kitchen. Entrances are narrow. Just make sure the aisle is wide enough for a person to walk through if the refrigerator is open. How wide does it need to be? That can depend on the refrigerator. If the refrigerator is an extra wide model the distance may need to be 48 inches. The narrowest door opening residential refrigerator is a side-by-side, counter depth model. Plan accordingly.

I know I harped on locating the refrigerator close to an entrance to the kitchen, however if there is a wall against the hinge side of the refrigerator there may be conflict in opening the refrigerator door against a wall. Often refrigerator doors need to be opened past 90 degrees to use the fruit and vegetable bins. Cleaning the refrigerator is also enhanced by opening the door past 90 degrees. Those shelves just don't want to come out unless the doors are WIDE open. There is also a problem with some refrigerators with their thick doors and the way they are hinged that require an inch or two clearance on the side to even open! Be safe and put a 12 or 15 inch cabinet between the wall and the hinge side of the refrigerator. This extra cabinet can also act as a landing space for items being pulled out of the refrigerator, (15 inches is recommended for a refrigerator landing area). Remember that side-by-side and French door models have hinges on both sides.

The refrigerator is not the only appliance with doors. Think about where the dishwasher and the oven are placed. Just like the refrigerator, both these appliances may have different door opening requirements. Some ranges have double ovens with a small oven on top of a bigger one. Even if one of these is currently used, plan for a more standard range because the appliance can easily be changed out and the next one may be a single cavity oven. Be on the safe side and plan for it.

If at all possible, don't open the oven into a major walk way where people that are not actively participating in cooking will be walking. Even though the kitchen should be just for the cooks people may still be walking through the area. My client's kitchen had an entrance from the dining room and another from the family room coming into the kitchen on one side and the entrance into the laundry which lead to the back yard on the opposite wall. Guess what was positioned in the string of counters between the doors; the range. The oven door is a trip point for those not actively cooking in the kitchen. The range is a place where pan handles can be caught on clothing and fall onto the floor.

The doors for the dishwasher and the oven need clear opening space in front of them. Make sure the doors do not conflict with other doors when opened. This includes cabinet doors and drawers. It is best to be able to walk between the open doors but this is not always possible. At a minimum allow a 42 inch aisle in front of the appliance as this will allow a person to stand in front of an open dishwasher or oven.

Another area to watch is placing the dishwasher too close to a corner. It is good to have standing room on both sides of the dishwasher when the door is open. Allow at least 21 inches for this.

If an appliance must be placed adjacent to a corner, use a spacer. The spacer will keep the appliance door from scraping against a not quite plumb wall. If the appliance is at right angles to another run of cabinets, the spacer will allow the door to open past the drawer faces and door pulls on the adjacent cabinets. I have seen an oven that could not open because of the knobs on the cabinet doors interfering. The owner had to remove all the knobs and one drawer that interfered to allow use of the oven. The spacers are also handy when placing cabinets at right angles to each other and a blind corner cabinet is used. The spacer prevents the same issues with the cabinets. Remember, spacers are your friends.

Sink area

The sink is the most used area in the kitchen. Even though I will cover sinks in the section on countertops I will mention here that they are an integral part of the work triangle no matter what work triangle is used. In a large kitchen there may be two or three work triangles. If this occurs try and keep the triangles from interfering with each other. Usually there is only one range in a kitchen unless it is a kosher kitchen. So both work triangles have to share the range but a second small sink can be added without taking up too much room. It is easier to reduce interference if the food preparation area is considered a part of the triangle instead of the refrigerator. But the refrigerator needs to be easily accessible to both without bumping into each other.

Multi-cook kitchen

More than one cook in the kitchen at one time creates its own challenges. Each cook will need their own area to work in. As mentioned above, both cooks will need to be able to access the sink. Two food preparation areas along with two sinks and a shared range will provide a workable arrangement. One person can be making a salad washing vegetables at the small sink while the other is prepping the main dish in another area.

If the kitchen is big enough, two full size sinks may be enjoyed. I do know of a person who has two full sinks in her kitchen with only a small amount of counter between them. This arrangement allows one person full access to a sink for cleanup or food preparation while the other is doing the same at a similar sink. This is a great setup if there are two dedicated cooks in the kitchen.

A food preparation area needs a minimum of 36 inches of counter frontage. If one of the preparation areas will be a baking area more length may be needed. There will be mixers and bowls and rolling pins and baking sheets that will be spread out. Plan on up to 54 inches of linear counter that is 24 inches deep. A baking area will also benefit from a lower (32 inch tall) base. This may be a very specialized area where the work triangle will look more like sink, baking area and oven. The oven is not usually considered part of the triangle because what goes into the oven does not need much attention until it is ready to come out. But baking cookies can be a more intense oven experience as they are often baked for a short time and require frequent checks for brownness.

Another possible food preparation area that might be included is a sit down area. If someone is in a wheelchair or just can't stand for long periods, a counter area at 30 or 32 inches tall might be very handy. Just make sure this person has access to one of the sinks.

Guest in the kitchen

There was a time when the kitchen was a closed off part of the house. Only intimate family members ventured there and even then it was the cook who was in charge and could shoo you out at any provocation – real or imagined. Horrors if a guest ever ventured into that territory which was never to be seen by visitors. That has all changed. The kitchen has come out of the closet so-to-speak. Now it is the gathering place for parties and the cook who use to slave away in their closed off room is now joining the party.

The challenge today is how to allow interaction with guest while keeping everyone safe from the hazards in the kitchen. Most of this is up to the proprietor of the house to make sure the dishwasher door is closed immediately after putting a dish in it and getting all the baking done before guest arrive. The main hazard is the stove top. Sometimes something is left simmering on the stove while the party is ensuing. The electric cook tops, especially the glass covered one can hold their heat for quite a while. A person may lean on it and get burned or maybe set a bag on the stove and have the plastic melt to the burner. My glass top range literature says to never put foil on the hot burner as it will not only melt to the burner but ruin the top in the process.

An island or a peninsula with a bar is a great solution. It defines the kitchen but allows visitors to sit and talk with the cook. Putting one of the main points of the work triangle (sink, stove or prep area) on the island or peninsula will insure that the cook has some good face time with visitors.

Putting the food prep area there will probably result in the most face time with visitors. Guest will often offer to help with tearing lettuce or cutting tomatoes when they can see what you are doing. If you want help in the kitchen, make sure the aisle is wide enough to accommodate two people. A 48 inch wide aisle is needed for two people to work comfortably. Make sure each person has their own work area.

If most of your social gatherings are catered, a more out-of-the-way kitchen may be desired. I have seen a house that accommodated both types of parties well. It had a very wide and long center hall like a dogtrot house. Against one side of the hall was the Family room with an entrance into this central hall. Against the other side of the hall was the formal dining room at the front of the house and the kitchen toward the back of the house. This allowed for easy mingling in and out of the kitchen for informal affairs. Formal dinner parties worked well in the same space by the use of sliding doors to close the kitchen and caterers off from the rest of the house.

A kitchen designer will ask you how you use your kitchen and what kind of entertaining you do so the best design can be developed for your use. The best time to bring in a designer is during the home planning stage, but if the house is already built, all is not lost. Much can still be done to make the space work better.

Access

I have mentioned before that the kitchen is the heart of the home; it is even in the book title. This does not mean every pathway in the house needs to run through it. But there are certain areas that benefit with direct or at least convenient access with the kitchen.

One is the outdoors. Often entertainment or grilling takes place outside. Both of these activities benefit from the kitchen being in close proximity. People are always moving back and forth between the outdoor deck and the kitchen for supplies or ice. I have seen a house where the kitchen was located at the front of the house and the owners placed their grill on the front porch when it was being used because the back deck was inconvenient. If the kitchen is unfortunately placed in your house and you do not want to go to the expense of moving the whole kitchen, consider an outdoor kitchen. These wonderful spaces accommodate not just a grill but a grill with burners, a small refrigerator, a self-contained ice maker and a sink. Remember to put in a prep area which could be part of the built in or could be a standalone table.

Pantry.

It would be great for everyone to have a pantry, and in fact everyone does. "What" you say? A pantry is just a place to store food items and some people have to use a wall and or base cabinet for this task. But most people who work in the kitchen much dream of a separate, large, walk-in pantry. Such a pantry is often located at the end of a run of cabinets or maybe located in an adjoining space such as laundry or utility room. Make sure such a pantry has adequate lighting to see what you have and vary the depth of the shelves. Deep shelves for large rarely used appliances and maybe baskets for things like potatoes and then shallow shelves for canned goods so you can actually see what you have and then some shelves in-between for storage of boxed goods. Sometimes you see these pantries located in the corner of a kitchen, intersecting two perpendicular cabinet runs. This can work out well, but I have seen kitchens, where the pantry in the corner cuts off what would have been a nice uninterrupted work space between the sink and the range. In this situation I would opt for moving the pantry. That work area between sink and stove is valuable real estate.

If the pantry needs to be somewhat smaller, consider a tall kitchen cabinet. These are the same depth as the base cabinets but go from floor to the same height as the wall cabinets. To make the tall kitchen cabinet more useful, make sure there are pull outs involved, either roll out shelves which will vary in width from 15 to 36 inches wide (of course in three inch increments) or a pull out system which can be as narrow as 6 inches. The whole objective is to be able to see what is actually in the pantry so nothing gets lost never to be seen until you move out of the house.

This brings us to the utility room or the laundry. The reason the laundry was originally located close to the kitchen was because the kitchen was such an active room and the idea was you could throw in a load of laundry while working in the kitchen thus saving steps. That is not the case anymore. Some people opt to put the laundry close to the bedrooms where the majority of the dirty clothes are generated. But even today, the logical placement of the laundry is close to plumbing so the expense of running long lines of water, sewer and extra vent pipes are avoided. So the laundry is best located close to a bathroom or the kitchen.

The utility room could also be termed the mechanical room as this is where the water heater and the electrical panel often reside. Sometimes this is located in the basement if one is used but other times it is located in a room with a door into the house, logistically close to the kitchen. I say logistically because a major use of hot water and electricity is in the kitchen. Having the two areas close to each other will save in plumbing and electrical cost, both expensive items. There are advantages to having the electrical panel in the house, if a circuit gets thrown (always seems to be during a thunderstorm) the box is easy to get to and the circuit flipped back on. I grew up in a house with the panel located on the side of the house and I remember my dad having to go out in the middle of a thunder storm with a flash light to find the circuit that had flipped.

That being said, I think the laundry/utility room combination is a good thing. And locating this area close to the kitchen is an even better idea.

Standard types of kitchens

In this section on traffic flow, I must cover the basic types of kitchens. Each type has different advantages and disadvantages.

The most basic type of kitchen is an In-Line kitchen. See the sketch below. This is where the kitchen cabinets and appliances are all against one wall as shown below. I lived in an apartment that had a kitchen like this. It was rather hard to use as there was not a lot of storage available. In my situation there was a wall that paralleled the cabinet wall. This wall had an opening on both ends so two people could run around the kitchen wall and not see each other. This set up is mainly used where space is at a premium.

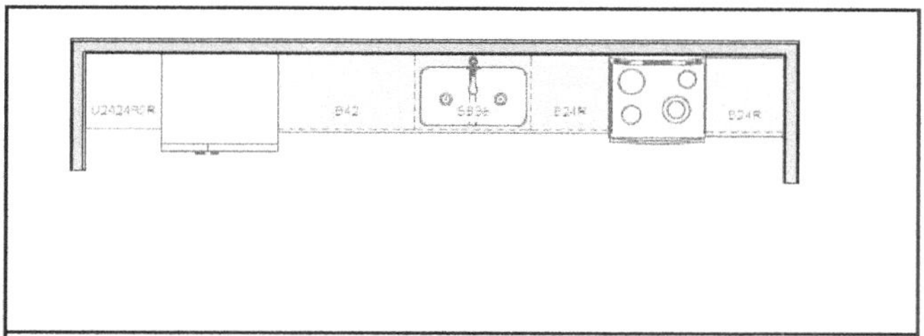

Inline Kitchen

Another problem inherent with this layout is the length required. To fit a 36 inch wide refrigerator, 36 inch wide sink base, 30 inch wide stove, 24 inch wide pantry, 24 inch wide dishwasher and all the work space and landing surfaces for the kitchen to work well you would need about 15 feet of length. That can translate into many steps back and forth while preparing the meal.

The second type of kitchen is a Galley Kitchen. See the sketch below. A galley kitchen is basically a hallway. There is an opening or doorway on each end so a person can pass straight through. Sometimes the opening is as shown in the picture, other time the openings may be straight through. But what distinguishes this kitchen from the in-line is the addition of cabinets on an opposite wall. I have also lived in a house with the setup as pictured. It seemed to have a lot of wasted space. In my case there was a very serviceable route around the kitchen so to create more counter and cabinet space I closed off one opening, creating a U Shaped kitchen.

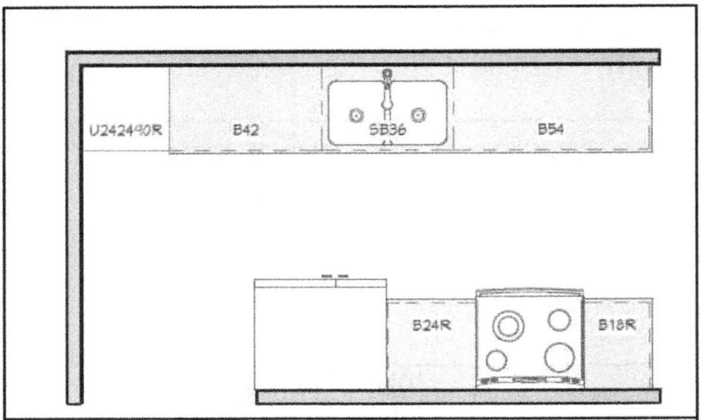

Galley Kitchen

Some Galley Kitchens will only have one entrance like in the apartment kitchen shown in the first chapter.

The third kitchen type is an L Shape, like the kitchen shown in the next figure. An L kitchen has cabinets on two walls but this time the second wall is adjacent to the first. This kitchen lends itself to being an eat-in kitchen where a kitchen table could easily be situated in the open area between the two runs of cabinets. An island would also be a wonderful addition to this style of kitchen so you can see it is very versatile. What I like about this version is that the range can be kept out of any major traffic pattern. By switching the sink and the range in the figure below, the range would be well protected.

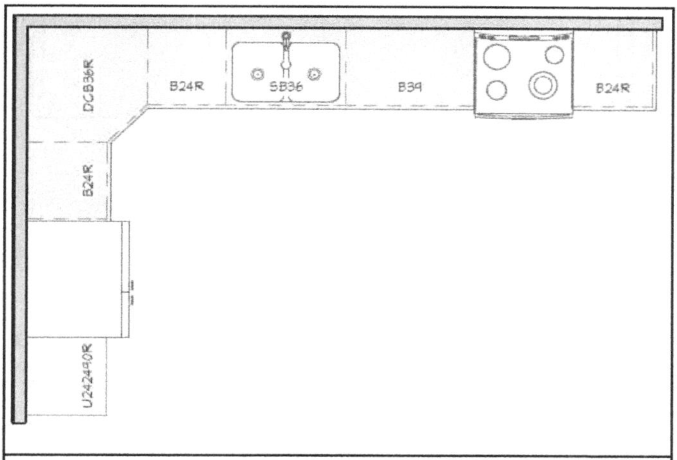

L Shape Kitchen

The fourth kitchen is a U Shape Kitchen. This is one of my personal favorites. Everything is within easy reach; there is a lot of counter surface on which to work and plenty of cabinetry for storage. This version of kitchen puts the cook in view of what is going on in the next room but keeps the kitchen out of the traffic pattern. But no matter how much I like this setup, I know this is not practical for all house designs.

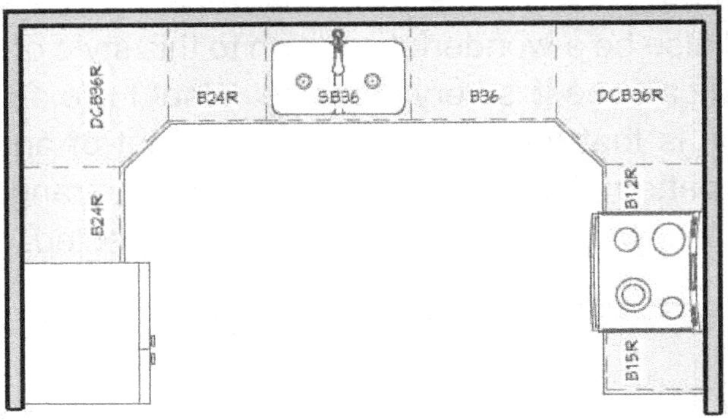

U Shape Kitchen

The fifth and final kitchen I will cover is the G Shape Kitchen. You can see this style kitchen on the facing page. This kitchen is very similar to the U shape kitchen but has an additional peninsula sticking out. In a way, this peninsula defines the territory. The cook is in their domain and all else stay out or enter in to help. The peninsula often serves as a bar where visitors can sit and watch the activities. This can become the equivalent of sitting at the breakfast table with a cup of coffee while visiting with a friend.

The bar can be at standard bar height or countertop height or even tabletop height.

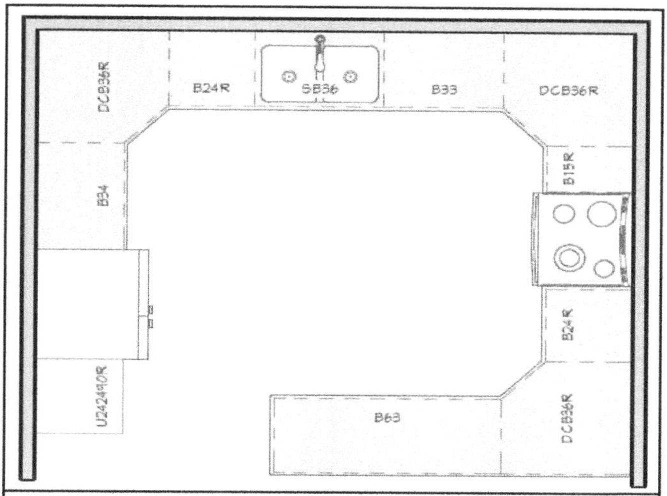

G Shape Kitchen

Each one of the above described kitchens has their own flow pattern concerning traffic from the rest of the house and also work flow for the kitchen activities. More than likely your home will lend itself to one or two possible kitchen types.

Go to https://akitchenyoulove.com/ch2 where you can decide on the work triangle that best fits your style of cooking and see more information.

Chapter 3
Storing Your Stuff

"He who has imagination without learning has wings but no feet."
—Joseph Joubert

Every good kitchen design has cabinets

I once read in a home design book that every good home design has a front door. Sometimes we take the simplest things for granted. So I wanted to get this out in the open. Your kitchen needs cabinets. Years ago there were not many cupboards in the kitchen; there was no need. All you had to store were a few plates and cups. Often these were stored right on the dining table. The pans were stacked close to the wood stove or hung on the wall. Food items were in the cellar and the dry goods were in a pie safe or some other container to keep the rodents out. And who needed serving dishes – those were for the wealthy – we served right from the cooking pan.

Times have changed considerably. We no longer have the "make do" attitude; we want all the gadgets that will make our quality of life better. We want the everyday dinnerware to use with the kids and the fancy dinnerware to use with the guests. We want the kid friendly plastic glasses and also the stemmed ware for special occasions. This includes all the serving dishes and silverware that goes with each set. Oh did I mention the proliferation of cookware available to the cook now days? That means we have to have a place to store everything and that place better be accessible. I think this is the real reason kitchens have gotten so big.

Then there is the food itself. Where does it go? Maybe you are lucky enough to have a large pantry but many homes don't or only have a very small, hard to access place that is used to store brooms, mops and vacuum. Oh and by the way food items that are accessed by moving out the brooms, mops and vacuum.

Often the kitchen is also expected to store non-food related items such as cleaning supplies and trash cans. Even though the mop, broom and vacuum may not actually end up in the kitchen slightly smaller items often do. Many times cleaning supplies are handily stored under the sink along with the trashcan. Some kitchens even have more than one trashcan: One for trash and one or more for recycling.

Then there are the pets. Usually their items (food dish, water dish) are found somewhere in the kitchen. What is a person to do? Where does it all go?

So although at first glance it may appear that picking out cabinets is all about picking out the style you like, it is so much more than that. It is about picking out your life style. It is about picking out accessibility. It is about how you want to live with your stuff.

Two basic types of cabinets

For years the most commonly used cabinets in the United States were "face frame" cabinets. More recently "frameless" or "European" cabinets have been gaining popularity.

Let me start with what the two have in common. They are both wooden boxes. They both come in the common dimensions. (See the section on spacing later). Both are available in any number of wood styles and colors depending on the manufacturer. Adjustable shelves are available with some manufacturers being more adjustable than others. Base cabinets can have a toe kick or sport furniture style feet. The backs may or may not be enclosed on either box, depending on the manufacturer.

The differences between frameless and framed cabinets can be striking with some people having a strong preference of one over the other.

The face frame is probably what you are more familiar with as it is what you grew up with or what your grandmother had in her kitchen. This is the standard box with a frame – like a picture frame but flat – around the front of the box. The inside opening of the frame is smaller than the inside of the box. Usually the bottom inner edge of the frame is flush with the bottom inner edge of the box but not always. The following picture shows an example of a face frame cabinet. Maybe you can see the hinge wrapping around the face frame. Is this what you have in your current kitchen? Most off-the-shelf cabinets will have face frames.

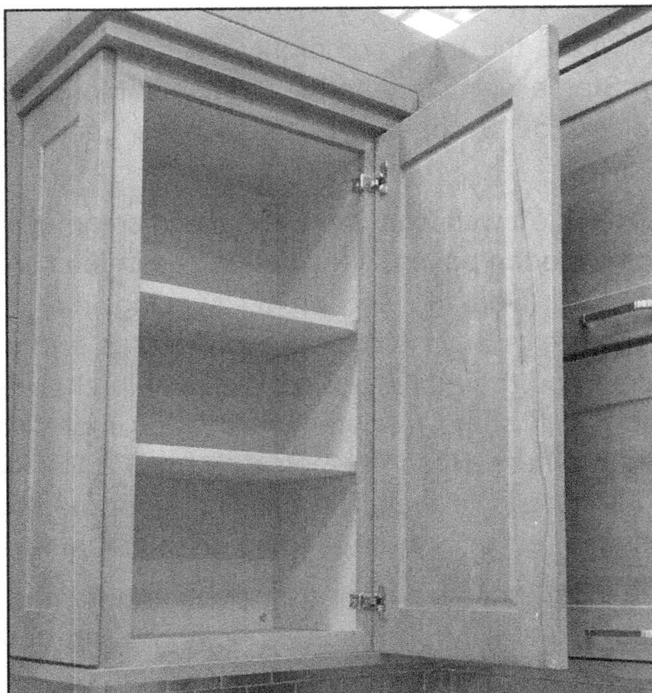

Face Frame Wall Cabinet

Photo by ND700/Shutterstock

I have seen cabinet boxes where the frame made a slight lip up from the bottom of the box interior. This might have been intentional or from sloppy workmanship. But this lip, even on the sides, can be a major irritation to some people as it makes the inside of the cabinet hard to clean and also hard to fit shelf paper. Ths lip can also catch large items as you are trying to get the items in and out of the cabinet.

For drawers, the lip around the opening can cut into the width of the drawer box by up to 3 inches. When you are trying to get every available fraction of an inch of storage from your kitchen, this can be a major disadvantage.

If face frames have such annoyances why use them? They do have their purpose. The frame lends strength and stiffness to the box. It is also easier to hide imperfect or out-of-plumb walls. The face frame cabinets also allow more choices in types of doors you can use. The doors can be inset which gives a clean, flush look to the cabinets. The doors can be overlaid on top of the frame where a stile (the exposed part of the face frame) may or may not show between the doors. Or the doors can be full overlaid on top of the frame where the doors almost touch each other when closed.

The most common door is the standard or partial overlaid door, not a full overlaid. Again this is what most off-the-shelf cabinets will have and is probably what you grew up with. Check your current cabinets. What type do you have? Below you will see an example of common overlaid doors, not a full overlay. Note how you can see the stile between the drawer and door fronts.Some of the larger well-known cabinet makers only deal in face frame cabinets, but many are starting to produce a frameless line of cabinets.

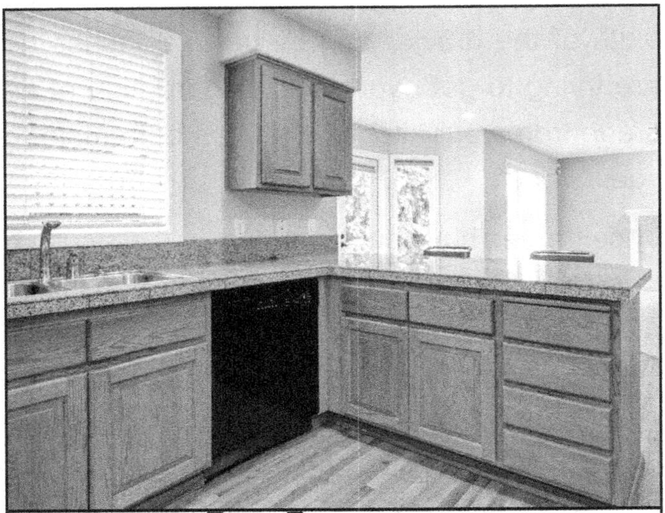

Face Frame Cabinets

Photo by Artazum/Shutterstock

The frameless, which is also referred to as the European style, is built without the frame. The box obtains its stiffness by other means. The following picture is an example of the frameless box during installation before the doors are attached. The side edges of the box are nicely finished but not trimmed out with a frame. Often these boxes will have a beautiful natural or wood stained finish and the doors will have the color that as requested when ordered. If you want the interior and outer edge to match the doors, be sure to specify that on your order. Most manufacturers can accomodate such a request for an extra cost. It may not be a problem to you to have the interiors not matching the door color. The doors will be full overlay so no edge or style will be showing when the doors are closed.

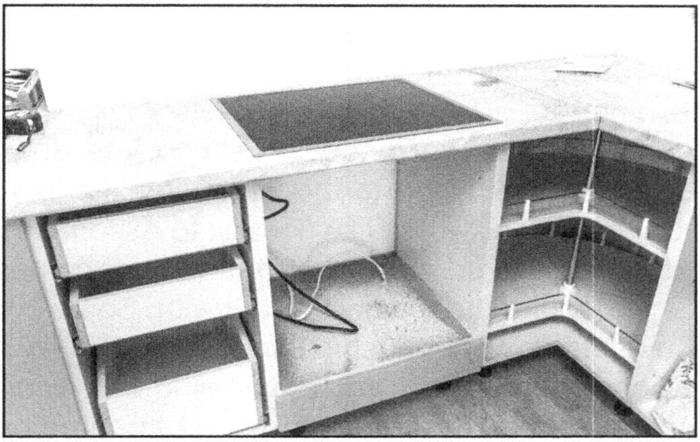

Frameless Cabinets

Photo by Garsya/Shutterstock

The full overlay may be a concern for some. But like the inset doors, the full overlay can create a nice, smooth,

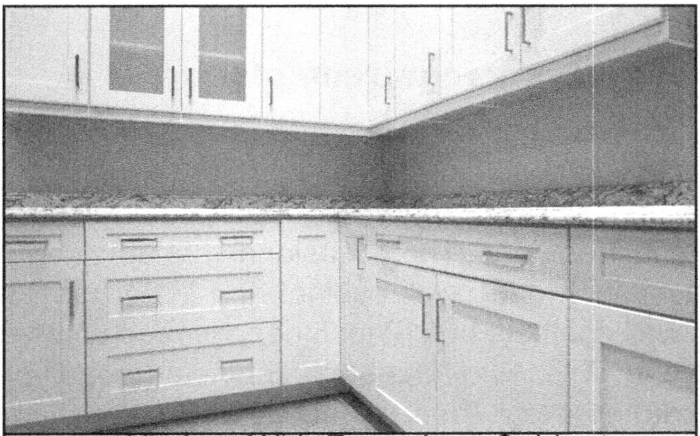

Kitchen With Frameless Cabinets

Photo by ND700/Shutterstock

clean look. See how nice and clean the surface looks in the picture above with the door and drawer fronts almost touching.

The Frameless or Euro style, as you might expect, originated in Europe. The Europeans have a different way of dealing with moving from house to house than we do. They take the kitchen cabinets with them. The true euro cabinets are made to be knocked down flat and easily shipped. Due to this characteristic this style is readily found online as RTA (Ready to Assemble) cabinets. I have ordered cabinets from several companies as RTA and found them easy to work with. Some companies have better workmanship than others and you tend to get what you pay for. If you are dealing with a contractor don't expect them to want to spend the time putting them together and any cost savings you might have on the product will be spent in labor by the contractor. But if you are willing to spend the weekend putting them together yourself, it can be a rewarding experience.

Unique spacing requirements

A standard has been established over the years that all cabinet manufacturers follow. Base (lower) cabinets are 24 inches deep and Wall (upper) cabinets are usually 12 inches deep. The occasional manufacturer might sell a 15 inch deep wall cabinet and IKEA has 13 inch deep wall cabinets but 12 inch deep is much more common in the US. All off-the-shelf cabinets (those you can load into your car from the store) and all semi-custom made cabinets come in widths of 3 inch increments starting at 9 inches wide. Some suppliers may go as low as 6 inch wide.

Why all this information about sizes of cabinets? There are two main reasons.

One is the doorways all these premade cabinets must fit through before they can be installed in a new kitchen. The wall cabinets should not have too much trouble, however keep in mind the length of the longest cabinet and any twist and turns or stair wells you have to snake it down. The base cabinets like the wall cabinets should fit through any doorway easily but they will be bigger and bulkier than the wall cabinets. Imagine carrying a base cabinet 54 inches long by 24 inches deep by 34 inches tall up a narrow flight of stairs with turns.

Secondly and more importantly is the length of the walls the cabinets will be going against. If the wall is 110 inches long, you will not be able to totally fill that wall with cabinets. The cabinet design will need to be somewhat shorter than the wall length.

If the cabinets are not captured on each end by an unmovable wall then you may be ok – as long as you don't mind a little wall sticking out past the cabinet. A good design for that 110 inch wall would be 108 inches of cabinet, with an extra 2 inches of wall space left over. However if the cabinet area has a wall on each end, having 2 inches of wall between the last cabinet and the wall will look funny. This is where a little strip of wood called a spacer or filler comes in handy. The contractor will space the cabinets against the wall leaving a gap between two cabinet sets for symmetry and then slip a spacer in the two gaps so the spacer is flush with the cabinet space. This will leave a gap when using full overlaid doors as the doors are sized for the cabinet not the cabinet with the spacer. The picture below shows how this might look on a full overlaid cabinet. See the matching spacer between the middle unit and the two side doors? If no spacer had been required, the doors would have a very small 1/8 inch gap between them.

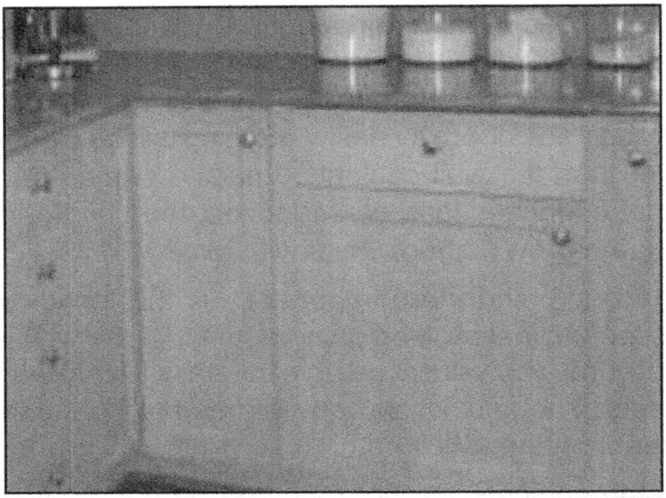

Base Cabinet With Spacers

Don't think of spacers as a nuisance but rather as a friend that can keep you out of trouble. Unless the cabinets are built in-place to fit, more than likely there will be gaps. Even if you measure the distance wall to wall and it comes out to 108 inches don't buy enough cabinet to precisely fill up the space. "Why" you ask? The cabinets are made fairly precisely with the use of electronic equipment in mass production and more than likely will be exactly 24 inches deep and exactly the width you requested but your house was not. I have yet to see a home builder who could build totally plumb and perpendicular walls. Even if the cabinets are not captured by a wall on one side, decide where you would like the cabinets to end and measure to that point acting like there is a wall there. That way if the wall on the other end is not plumb and you have to shim the cabinet away from the wall some you will be OK on the open end. If you are not real concerned about where the cabinet ends up – go for it.

Another useful place for spacers is at corners whether the corner is another cabinet or a wall. A spacer will allow the door or drawer to open without hitting a knob or handle on an adjacent cabinet or scraping the wall.

The height of the matter

There are also standard heights for kitchen cabinets. In general base cabinets are built 34.5 inches tall. Adding a standard 1.5 inch thick countertop brings the assembly top surface to 36 inches above the floor which is a good work surface height for the average person standing straight up. If you are into making pastries or breads you may want a section that is shorter with a finished height of 32 inches. This is a good height for the average person to roll out dough or punch down bread and accounts for leaning over the work surface to put weight on the dough or roller. There may be other reasons you want a different height for a counter. Some people want to raise the dishwasher to make it easier to load and unload. The same may apply to an oven where a person may want a built-in oven at eye level while someone else will want it just under the counter to allow more counter space.

Then there are microwave ovens. It can be mounted in the base cabinet or it could be mounted in a wall cabinet or it could go somewhere in between. Some like the microwave as part of the vent hood for the range but this is too high for many people.

There is no right or wrong mounting position but try and keep the bottom of the microwave 54 inches or less above the floor. Higher than that and it is hard for the average height person to see what is going on and there is risk of spilling hot items on themselves.

If you plan on selling the home in the next 5 years stick with what the average person will be expecting in a house of your caliber. If you want to live in the home for a long time, go with what fits you and feels comfortable to you.

Then there are tall cabinets. These are the ones that run from floor to ceiling. Be sure to measure your ceiling height to make sure the unit will actually fit in the space. And you thought the base units were hard to get in the house! These tall utility cabinets come with the toe kick unattached otherwise you would never be able to install them. Installation is the tricky part. Remember your geometry in school? Think of a right triangle. This is the one with a 90 degree corner. This utility cabinet will be in each of these side positions at some point. When you bring it in the house it will be laying down on its side. When you stand it up it will be the vertical side but to get to this position it has to become the hypotenuse – the long side of the triangle.

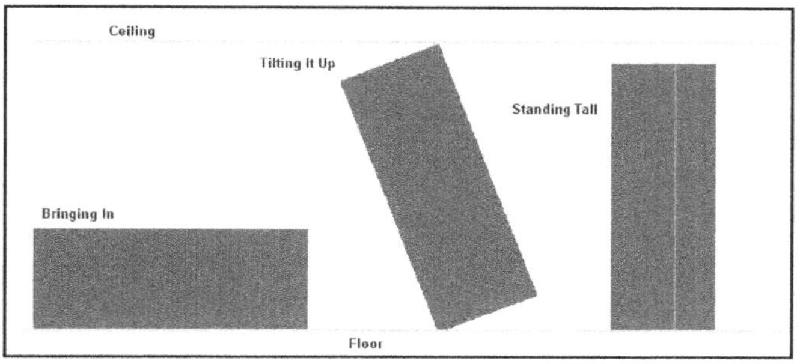

Tall Cabinet Height Requirement

As you stand it up you will note a conflict with the ceiling unless you have very high ceilings. The only way to get this bugger to stand up with a standard ceiling is to remove the toe kick. That 4 inches will make all the difference in the world and even then it will be tight. After you finally get that unit vertical put the toe kick where the unit will finally rest then carefully (with two people or more) raise the cabinet onto the toe kick. This is also why you want the ceiling height to actually be a little taller than the cabinets and then use crown molding or a trim piece to cover the gap between cabinet and ceiling.

You can do so much more with cabinets than the standard wall cabinets hung above the base cabinets. Think outside the box. It is also possible to mix and match cabinets to get the look you want. By stacking two wall cabinets on top of a toe kick made from 2x4s you can have a real nice book case as shown in the next picture.

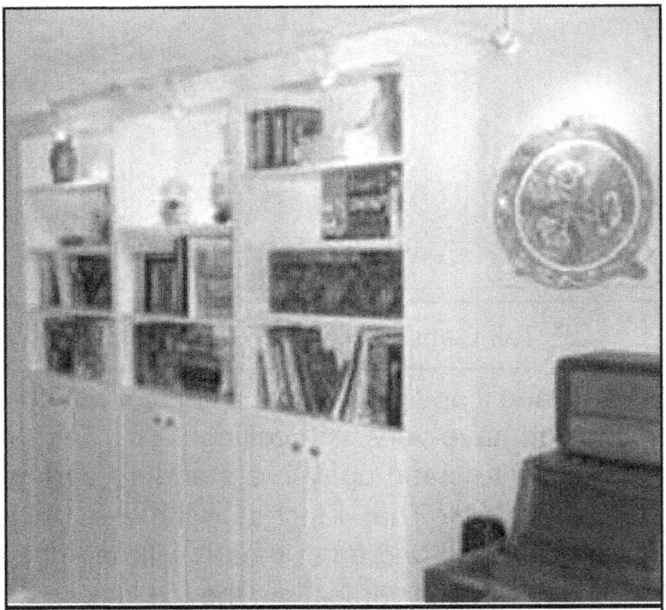

Face Frame Wall Cabinet

Cabinets can be ordered with or without doors. Six wall cabinets were used in the bookcase above. Three were ordered with doors and three without.

What comes with your cabinets

Hopefully your base and wall cabinets will have adjustable shelves. The Euro style frameless cabinets have drilled holes in the sides to allow multiple adjustable shelves at many heights. The holes are also used to mount the hinges and drawer slides. Although you will initially set your heights based on what you put in the cabinet from the start and never move them after that it is still very handy to have the adjustable shelves. This lends a custom feel to the cabinets as you load them up. This feature became so popular that the companies building the face frame cabinets followed suit and also provide adjustable shelves in some of their cabinets. It was not all that long ago that I had to be careful when buying cabinets to make sure the shelves were adjustable. Now it is almost taken for granted that they are adjustable. There is still one advantage with the frameless cabinets concerning shelves – the shelves are much easier to slide in and out: there is no face frame to get in the way.

Now comes the dilemma of shelves versus drawers. I have found drawers to be handier than doors when it comes to base units. However drawers are more expensive. Face it, they are harder to make, require more wood and more hardware. But they are often worth it. I have also used roll out shelves in base cabinets to allow access to the back of the shelf and to store heavier items where I can more easily reach them. If you are concerned with price, check with your cabinet supplier to see which is more economical, drawers or roll out shelves. Different cabinet makers may price one higher than the other and it may not always be the drawers.

Pantries are also much more useful with drawers. If you want the look of doors but the convenience of drawers, use roll out shelves as in the pantry shown in the following figure.

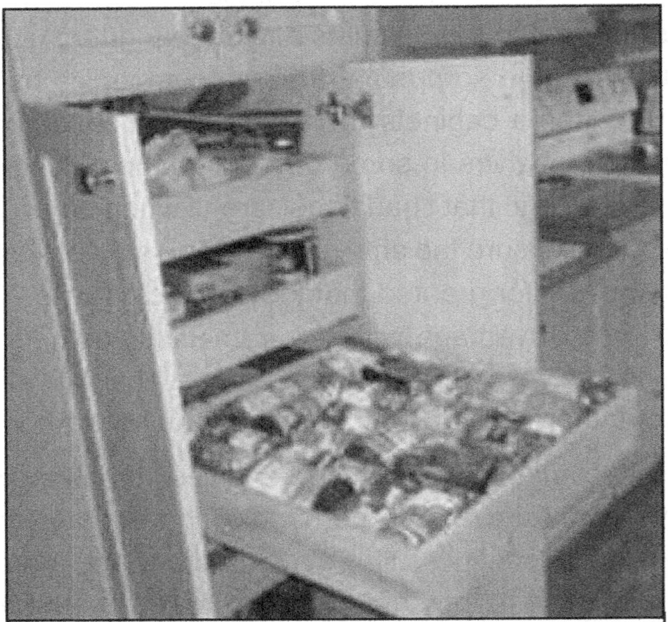

Pantry With Drawers

Here all the cans are on their side with the labels facing up. This makes it easy to see what is in the pantry and all of the space gets used. The very sides of the cabinet are not usable because of the thickness of the sides of the drawers and the mounting of the hinges and glides, but I could argue that more of the space in the cabinet is used because items do not get lost in the black hole at the back of a two foot deep shelf never to be seen again. Because the example is a frameless cabinet with undermount slides, there's not too much space wasted – just the thickness of the drawer sides and a small gap.

Something to watch out for on the lower cost cabinets is the use of half shelves. Often you have to hunt for this bit in the literature if you are buying on line as they really do not want to advertise that the buyer will be getting a short shelf. This is a shelf that comes with the base cabinet that is only one foot deep not the whole depth of the base unit. This is difficult to work with because the front of the shelf is a foot back from the front of the cabinet.

The more expensive and often the mid-range price cabinets will have the heavy duty Blum brand soft-close drawer slides and door hinges. I have to say that I really like the soft close drawer slides. They slide so smoothly, feel so substantial and close so easily. I am still not so sure about the soft-close hinges. I am trying both the standard and the soft-close in my laundry room cabinets and I keep finding myself trying to make the soft-close doors close faster. I guess they are not just soft close but slow close. It doesn't help to force them, rather it works best to just "bump" them in the right direction and let them close themselves.

Material choices

No matter how good the plumbing something invariably happens and the drain or a hose fitting will come loose and spill water under the sink. You do not want a base cabinet that will start to blister and decompose after it gets damp. Do not get a box made from Masonite or Melamine; these products are known to fall apart in water. MDF board (MDF stands for Medium Density Fiber) is a popular item among carpenters because it is easy to cut and easy to paint but like the Masonite it will delaminate when wet. The MDF is ok for the door fronts as it is a stable product and so is less likely to warp, shrink and expand with temperature and humidity changes, just don't let it sit in water. Melamine is just a plastic coating over MDF material. For the cabinet box, especially sink bases, insist on plywood or solid wood. The plywood is the more common for the box.

Most manufacturers produce several price (quality) levels of their products. The lower cost version will usually be made with the undesirable product. Spend the extra money for a better product that will last you many years. This is not an item you will want to change out in a couple of years because the bottom rotted out.

Remember that unlike the cabinet box, the drawer fronts and doors are often made from solid wood and wood is affected by humidity. Wood can swell in humid times of years and shrink in dryer times especially in the first year as it acclimatizes to its new environment. The doors themselves may look warped or don't appear to shut flat. This is more prevalent in solid wood doors or doors with wide wood stiles and rails. The center panel may be made from a different material and often 'floats' between the stiles and rails. This will allow for expansion and contraction of the wood used without so much warpage.

So don't panic if your doors do not lay absolutely flat. Give it several months to a year to flatten out.

There are a number of woods to choose from. The most popular is Oak which has a strong grain that takes almost any stain color. Oak also comes in White Oak and

Red Oak. If you want a dark or reddish stain go with the Red Oak for something a little lighter use the White Oak. But remember the grain in Oak really stands out and will come through in the stain and sometimes in the paint.

Another popular wood is Cherry that has a natural reddish color somewhat deeper than the Oak. Hickory is another popular wood with a strong brown color and many natural markings. If you want something lighter, Birch is a very white wood that stains easily. One of my favorites is Ash which is also rather white but what I like about it is the very little grain that shows through. Ash also readily takes stains and is easy to paint. Maple is another wood that has light graining and is often used.

Of course there are many other exotic woods which could be used when custom made cabinets are used but the ones mentioned above are what will be most common from the ‘well known’ manufacturers. But whichever wood is used, be aware that the look of the finish may change with time as the wood ages and UV light affects it. There may also be small imperfections in the wood due to “bird pecks” or wormholes. The way the tree grew and the wood cut may expose knots and other blemishes. If a smoother more consistent look is desired then maybe another material should be used.

Other possible materials are veneers which are thinly sliced sheets of wood that are attached to a panel. This looks like real wood but has a more consistent grain and color. Thermofoil is another interesting material/process. Thermofoil is created from a thin layer of PVC film that is shaped and glued to MDF (remember that from above?) and then heat and pressure is applied to seal it to the surface. The surface becomes seamless and covers the whole panel. This is great for wear and cleaning. A third alternative to the wood is a laminated acrylic that is applied to a core material and it gives a fashion forward look to the cabinet.

I have also seen metal used for doors and drawers. This is a very industrial look that may work well for an inner city loft. I am not real fond of metal drawer boxes. The ones I have seen are noisy to use and eventually rust as the protective coating gets scraped off.

Abundance of door styles

I have already mentioned the flat slab doors and the stiles and rails with an inset panel. The full overlay, standard overlay and inset have also been mentioned above. We are now talking about looks. I know this is a book about function but this is a needed topic. Choosing a door style is where most people get so confused because the choices are so many.

Look at the pictures you have clipped or the file of photos you have from Pinterest. Look at the overall style you are gravitating towards. Is it fancy with a lot of scroll work and curves or is it cleaner almost industrial? Or maybe it falls in between. If you have not chosen the flat modern or industrial look you have picked one of the paneled doors. Now is it a raised panel or a recessed panel?

A raised panel has the center panel that is raised up but no higher than the outside stiles and rails. These doors and drawer fronts can get pretty fancy with various layers and steps between the edge pieces and the inner panel. You may also see the upper rail with an arch or other fancy attributes.

A recessed panel is when the middle panel is sunken or inset from the outside edge. The edges themselves may be of varying widths. These doors are usually simpler in looks to the raised panel. The stiles and rails may have a sharp clean line down to the panel or they may have an angled slope to the panel. There may also be a third stile in the middle but that is as fancy as it gets. I have seen a few that trim out the edge of the stile and rails with a fancier molding as it heads down to the panel. The drawer fronts may be made of a single flat panel or they may have the stiles and rails to match the doors.

Doors don't have to swing side to side. For a more modern flare or even an older looking elegance consider the doors that open upward. They can add interest when paired with the standard swing doors.

For more interest and to display items, glass panels in the doors can be beneficial. They don't have to be clear but can be made of any number of textured glasses or even stained or beveled glass.

After you settle on a door style you get to make another choice. There is the option of wood stain, paint or going with one of the fused overlays. A lot of people have panic attacks at the thought of painting a beautiful piece of wood. Don't be upset if you really like wood but really want paint. Many of the painted versions are made from the wood that would not quite make a good stained piece.

All these doors do the same thing so this is where you get to make your creative statement for your kitchen. Unlike the cabinets themselves, the doors and drawer fronts can be changed out and updated several years later if you get tired of them. It won't be cheap to do but it won't cost as much as changing out all of the cabinets.

What goes in those beautiful cabinets? There are all kinds of handy inserts that can really help you get the most use out of your cabinets. Most all cabinet manufacturers can provide slide out shelves for their base cabinets. These are handy for all types of situations and it doesn't have to be just one or two shelves for a base unit. Request extra sliding shelves to store lids flat on a shelf not requiring much height. Use a slide out shelf up high in the base cabinet to store those 50 bottles of spices, lying down so the labels can be read from above.

A concealed trash can or even a combination trash can and recycle bin can come in handy. Now the trash can is coming out from under the kitchen sink and getting its own space in a pull out cabinet. Sometimes two are in the same pull out drawer.

Pots and pans can be stored in a deep drawer close to the range. Or the drawers may actually be slide out shelves that are hidden behind doors. There are also slide out racks that can hang pans on one side and lids on the other.

A divider for silverware may lay flat in a shallow drawer or stand tall in a deep drawer. There are also sliders for double stacking the silverware in a drawer. When the drawer is open the top tray is seen, but push it back and out of the way and a deeper second layer is revealed. Cutting boards can also be stored like this with the board being above the drawer but camouflaged with the drawer face when closed. A knife drawer can keep the knives organized and sharp and off the counter.

How about storing the dishes in a lower drawer? There are dividers or pegs that can be inserted in the drawer at strategic places to keep the dishes from moving around and hitting each other.

If there is room for a very small 6 inch wide base unit, that is wide enough to store spices, oils and vinegars for cooking. Other specialty cabinets may include a wine rack or a hanging rack for stem ware.

The spices can be stored in drawers flat or tilted or in wall cabinets. There are also units that mount on the inside of a wall cabinet door. Any of these items can make the spices easy to see and find.

Don't forget a divider to stand your cookie sheets for easy access. This would usually go in a base cabinet because the sheets are often deeper than 12 inches.

The infamous corner cabinets with their dark deep recesses often benefit with the addition of a Lazy Susan. There are cabinets that fit into corners that are not Lazy Susan cabinets, these are called blind corner cabinets. A traditional Lazy Susan will not fit in that type of cabinet. However there are products that will work in such cabinets, making the back recess of that cabinet accessible. See the picture below for an example of a half moon Lazy Susan.

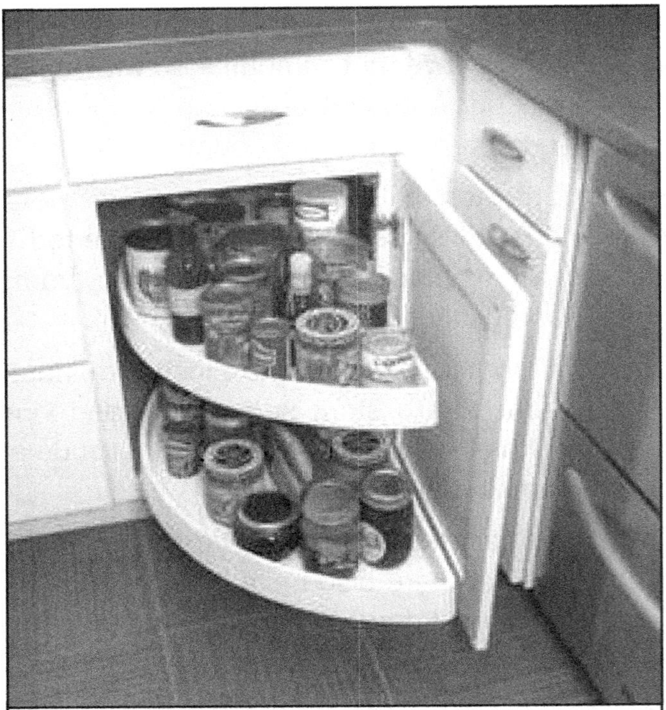

Half-Moon Lazy Susan

Often these additions are available from the cabinet company. For those smaller companies that may not be able to provide all the bells and whistles there are after-market products that can be purchased from one of the big box stores or a bed and bath store.

Stock vs. semi-custom vs. custom vs. mail order

There are a number of ways to buy cabinets. They can be bought right off the shelf at a big box store or some lumber yards. These are stock cabinets and are usually limited in style and sizes. They may be adequate if a small cabin or rental property needs cabinets but they will not satisfy most people. The workmanship on these cabinets is often on the low quality side. Don't expect these to last or perform like a better quality product. If used in rental housing, expect the drawers to break and doors to come off or warp. They may be a constant irritation. However for a vacation cabin that is lightly used this may fit the bill. They are usually the least expensive of the cabinet choices.

The semi-custom cabinets can also be obtained at the big box stores along with various cabinet shops. These are ordered and delivered directly to the work site. Expect delivery to take 4-8 weeks. There are usually specific sizes in which the cabinets can be ordered but the options are much broader than the stock cabinets. Often various inserts like Lazy Susan are available. The prices for these can vary substantially depending on the manufacturer. Each manufacturer will also have different options and inserts available for their cabinets at a price of course. Semi-custom cabinets also come in many choices for finishes and wood species. These manufacturers often offer various versions of their cabinets. They will have a lower end and a higher end. The higher end will often have more option choices than the lower end. Semi-custom cabinets are the most common cabinet bought.

Some manufacturers of the semi-custom cabinets can vary the sizes of their cabinets to a more custom fit. The lines are getting blurred between the semi-custom and custom cabinets.

A custom cabinet is just that, custom cabinetry. A craftsman or carpenter will measure your space; using those dimensions they will create the pieces that will fit your home. Other pieces in the home may also be built to keep the style and paint or stain consistent throughout the home. The craftsman is only limited by his imagination and the products that are available to him. The wood will often be oak, birch, or whatever is common to the location but they are able to order more exotic pieces to use. The highly skilled craftsman can mix a stain special for the project so the exact shading desired is obtained. Often these cabinets will be built in place so they fit the room like a glove and no spacers are needed to hide gaps. Sounds good doesn't it? Of course these will cost more than the semi-custom but unless the more exotic woods and specialty stains are chosen the pricing may not be that much more. So if you have real picky taste, this may be the way to go.

The last option is mail order. Many people do this. I have ordered several cabinets online and this works well if you are not too picky. One company sent me the taller 36 inch cabinets for the master bathroom vanity instead of the standard lower height I ordered but I did not realize it until we had installed it and I noticed the sink seemed high. It actually worked well in the situation and we decide to keep this more expensive vanity.

The mail order cabinets are often RTA (Ready to Assemble). This means that the buyer or contractor will be assembling the cabinets. They are often frameless cabinets and require a minimum amount of tools to assemble. Some go together easier than others. I have been very impressed with the products I have received. I have been able to find real wood cabinets and the pricing is usually less than the quality semi-custom. A few companies ship their cabinets already assembled. These cabinets may take 6 – 8 weeks to arrive at the job site and then it will take several days to put all the kitchen cabinets together.

Universal design and accessibility

More and more designs and products are geared toward the universal design concept. First let me clarify the difference between universal design and accessibility. Universal design is geared to make the area more usable and functional for people no matter their size, age or ability. This concept is what brought us the levered handled door knobs and the levered sink controls. Accessible design is geared more to the particular requirements of a specific person with unusual characteristics and needs. In other words, everyone benefits from universal design while a few benefit from accessible design. Sometimes what may start out as accessible design will end up as universal design for example the placement of wall ovens. Ovens traditionally were either located at base cabinet height as in under a range top or double stacked in a tall cabinet. To make the ovens more accessible to a person sitting in a wheel chair the ovens were unstacked and placed side by side at a height that is within easy reach of a seated person. Nowadays it is not uncommon to see that placement in a standard home because it is just a much easier height for a standing person to access: no bending and lifting.

Universal design is a great approach to design as it makes a space so much easier to use for all. Sometimes in our lives we may experience some sort of disability which will highlight the benefit of universal design. Think of a broken arm and how much easier it is to open a lever handle door with your injured arm while carrying items in your good hand. So read this section with the idea that some of these items may currently be labeled as accessible design but may be found in the universal design before too long.

Do you know someone who has trouble hearing in a noisy environment? Although some people are born with hearing problems or obtain such problems through illness or accident, this is a common occurrence as we age. Good design can help reduce hearing problems associated with loss of frequency range or with ringing in the ears. Just reducing the reverberation of sound by selecting sound-absorbing materials for walls, floors and window treatments can help. Also the use of quiet appliances and ventilation equipment can help.

The big category that most people think of when they think of accessible design is physical mobility. A person does not have to be in a wheel chair to benefit from mobility considerations. Think of a person with arthritis or on crutches due to a broken leg or how about a pregnant woman. Each of these has different mobility issues that could benefit from a little thoughtful planning. Considerations include; width of passage ways, selection of drawer pulls, location and ease of use of controls.

A person's height can be important in accessible design. This category is listed under accessible design because it is so personal. I have seen some people who are very tall and would benefit from extra tall base cabinets such as Julia Childs who at 6'2" had 38 inch tall base cabinets instead of the standard 36 inch. Then at the other end of the standard adult scale of 4'11" for a short woman (even though I know people who are shorter) who would benefit from shorter cabinets. However, with short people there are other options such as step stools or even toe kicks that could be pulled out to provide a step. Often more than one person uses the space and so various heights must be accommodated. Providing multiple height work surfaces in the kitchen allows accommodation for most every person who may use the space.

Arm reach must also be mentioned here as all plugs and switches must be accessible to those using the space. A person seated at the standard 25 inch deep kitchen counter may be able to reach the wall surface up to 44 inches above the floor. Plugs and switches above this height would potentially be unusable by such a person.

I touched on width of passage ways earlier when I was talking about physical mobility, but what is considered a good size? A 32 inch clear space is considered acceptable for a door opening, but remember if there is a door installed and not just an opening, that opening will be narrower (the door takes up some of the space, even when full open) so use a 34 inch door to obtain the 32 inch min. clear space.

This leads right into floor space. For accessibility (think wheelchair) a 5 foot minimum radius is needed in which to turn a wheelchair around. Clear space is also required around each appliance and down walkways. There are access standards published by the International Code Council (ICC/A117.1) that describe the minimum clear space required in all such area. If there is a wheelchair involved, the use of a professional kitchen designer will be well worth the expense, even if only to look over your own designs to make sure everything is accessible.

Looking at the kitchen you are in now, have you considered how you might get to the kitchen sink if you were in a wheelchair? There are various configurations to allow a person in such a situation to get close to the sink. They all have to do with providing knee space. A 36 inch wide area is required to comfortably accommodate a wheelchair and that is the same width as the average sink base. Most accessibility versions involve some method of opening up the area below the sink to allow a chair to roll into the space. A lower sink base is also desirable.

If you look at many brochures on kitchen cabinets you will see some cabinets with extra tall toe clearance. These may be 6 inches tall (standard toe clearance is 3.5 to 4 inches) and will also be extra deep. This is to accommodate the foot rest on a wheelchair. Although this gets the chair a little closer to the cabinet it still does not allow the person to easily work at the counter. Other accommodations must be made such as a lower pull out work surface that a seated person can get under.

Another big area for accessibility are the appliances themselves. The ovens were mentioned above but the dishwasher is another item that will benefit with being raised for accessibility. How about the microwave? It needs to be at a height that a person can pull hot items from with ease and below eye level. The standard reach for a wheelchair bound person is considered 15 inches from the floor up to 48 inches above the floor.

To see colored versions of the above pictures and a video on frameless vs. face framed cabinets check out https://akitchenyoulove.com/ch3

Chapter 4
Topping Your Cabinets

"A rock pile ceases to be a rock pile the moment a single man contemplates it, bearing within him the image of a cathedral."

—Antoine de Saint-Exupery

History of countertops

What do you use to top those cabinets? There are many materials available for your countertops. Each decade has their "New" material that later falls out of favor. Up through the early 1900s people did not even have counters as we know them. They had wood tables for work surfaces, often the same tables used for eating around. So of course these had wood tops. As the years went by, wood was used for counter tops out of habit. But the wood started falling out of favor because of the focus on disease and bacteria. People realized that the wood was hard to keep clean or even see if it was clean, so tile was introduced as the new material of choice for the hard working counters. The tiles were kept very tight to each other to keep the grout lines small (which were hard to clean) and the tile edges close due to their sharp nature (unlike current tiles).

In the roaring 20's more women of the house were doing the cooking with less servants helping out. More prepared foods were becoming available and storage was needed. This created a need for cabinetry in the kitchen. People were building cabinets in their home and some were lucky enough to afford to order the new pre-made modular cabinets of the time. The countertop was still primarily tile but the colors were getting brighter and the shapes were getting more interesting. You may be wondering about marble countertops. Many people think of marble when they think of the 20s. Yes marble was often used for working pastries or candy making. Marble's cool, smooth surface was ideal for this. The 20's also saw zinc being used on some items but this was rare and had limited use. If the budget was really tight during this time frame, a left over piece of floor linoleum may also have made its way to the countertop position.

The 30s saw the development of new materials for the countertop. Melamine and the precursor of Formica came on the market. But this was expensive especially during the depression years and so tile was still the common material.

The 40s saw a few improvements as the nation struggled to get back on its feet. Tile was still the main material with the hex tiles becoming the most popular design during this time. Square tiles, when used, were often laid in more interesting patterns such as at a diagonal to create a diamond pattern or with smaller squares of contrasting colors. The linoleum product which became Formica was still being used and often seen with a plain metal edging.

In the 50s, tile is still the main material but Formica (a laminate) is gaining popularity. With the soldiers coming home from the war and the nation rejoicing they were ready for a little fun. During this time, many interesting colors and designs were introduced, making the Formica product hard to resist. And of course the metal edging has now become a main stay. Speaking of metal, by this time stainless-steel has become a popular alternative to the other metals previously used in the kitchens. Another infamous countertop material of the time is still linoleum flooring. It was not that common but mainly used because it is the least expensive way to go.

If you are trying to build a historic kitchen you are in luck. Most of the materials mentioned above are still available, however you might want to stay away from the linoleum flooring. But many of the 'historical' kitchens today may have a more extensive use of marble along with soapstone, slate or granite. Stones were not commonly used for countertops in the past because they were hard to cut, transport and hone to a smooth surface. The stones also left little holes and imperfections for food particles to get into which would harbor and promote bacterial growth.

The 60s were a booming time for the laminate industry. If you have a midcentury home and want it to look midcentury, use a laminate with a metal edging and you can't go wrong. Another 60s product that no one knows about any more was called Lusterock. It was basically an indestructible material made from quartz chips, Mother of Pearl, Italian quartz, rocks and shells (along with anything else that fell in the mixture) imbedded in a polyester resin. Too bad that product is no longer available, it sounds awesome.

What about more modern times? (Were the 70s modern?) The 70s – any of you remember them? The brands Formica and Wilsonart produced most of the countertops of that age. Some of these were in bright colors to contrast and compliment the harvest gold and avocado green colored appliances that were popular at the time. But still the colors choices only amounted to a dozen or so.

The 80s saw a lot of new materials come into use. Synthetic materials such as solid acrylic surfacing had the advantage of being molded in a single seamless piece including the sink and backsplash. The laminate countertops were losing their top standing.

From the 90s until today many new materials have entered the market. Some are not so new but are being used in a new way. Concrete is one of those materials. I guess metal can also qualify as a manmade product that has taken over as a surface material. The list for metals includes not only zinc like we saw in the earlier kitchens but also includes stainless steel, copper, aluminum and even pewter. Of course solid surfacing is still available. One brand that most people recognize is Corian. Quartz, another manmade product, is also popular at the present time. Like quartz, there are other products that are resin based such as Vetrazzo which is a recycled glass product in a resin. A similar product is IceStone which is 100% recycled glass in a cement substrate. How about paper imbedded in resin? I know it sounds weird but “PaperStone", "Squak Mountain Stone" (yes, that's spelled correctly), and "EcoTop" are three paper countertops manufactures. It's a great way to go if you are ecologically minded.

For the more right out of the ground products try granite. The recent years have seen granite really taking off as a countertop material. As of the mid 2010s Granite is the most popular countertop material. Guess what is in second? Our old friend laminates such as Formica or Wilsonart. But now the laminates have hundreds of colors and patterns to choose from. For third place, look to quartz.

Getting back to stone, this is the first time stone has really been popular as a kitchen counters. Soapstone was used regionally in the East in the 50s but nothing like the way granite is being used today. Granite is not the only popular stone. There is a whole list of natural surfaces to choose from: Marble, travertine, Limestone, Soapstone, Quartzite and Onyx.

Another natural product that is back again is wood. Wood as butcher block, wood as furniture grade plywood and all kinds of exotic woods in-between. Some companies make their countertops from reclaimed wood from old barns, warehouses, commercial buildings and wine vats. If you are interested in reclaimed wood check into "Craft-Art" or "Endurawood"

Cost

Which product is the most economical? That is a hard one. Prices vary considerably from year to year and from product to product. Currently quartz is more expensive than granite but several years ago when the cost of crude oil was cheaper (being a major component in the manufacture of quartz countertops), quartz was less expensive than granite. First decide what material is really desired then shop around for the best price. If the desired price cannot be found, choose a different product that has many of the qualities liked in the first choice and shop again. If price is the major factor in choice, laminate may be the way to go. Even the highest quality laminate can be less expensive than the lowest quality quartz or granite. There is a reason laminates are the second most popular countertop material.

I really don't want to list prices here because they will be outdated by the time this is printed. Also each product comes in a range of cost. Usually the lower end of the range is based on popularity (least popular being less expensive), quality and thickness of the particular item. However I can list the products from least expensive to most expensive based on their lowest price as of this writing. That list is as follows: Laminate, Tile, Butcher Block, Granite, Solid Surfacing, Recycled Glass, Quartz, Marble, Stainless Steel, Soapstone, Concrete, Paper Composite. Even this list may vary depending on location. I have seen Stainless Steel and Solid Surfacing cheaper than Granite so decide what you really want then shop around. If you can't find what you want in your price range go to your second choice. Don't pick something from the above list as a compromise because of cost right from the start; you may be cheating yourself from what you really want when it is in your budget at your location.

For budgeting purposes expect to spend from $20 to $250 per square foot of counter needed. Yes consider the kitchen sink and any other sinks as counter top space as they do have a rim of counter around them and have the added expense of cutting out the hole.

Maintenance

Something to consider when picking a countertop material is maintenance and general cleaning. When I say general cleaning, I am thinking bacterial growth or lack of it which is what is desired. Some materials are more easily cleaned than others. The surfaces that are nonporous will not support bacterial growth and will clean up easily. Some surfaces such as natural stones are either soft like Marble or porous like Granite and Concrete which will collect food particles in the pores promoting bacterial growth. These can be sealed but even then Marble can still stain and frequent resealing may get tiresome. Remember the Paper Composite countertop? Well it also requires maintenance and more often than most other countertops. Wood is another product that harbors bacteria and needs tender loving care to keep it in good shape.

Which are the nonporous surfaces? Well our old stand-by Laminate is one. Tile can also be nonporous however the grout is not and the grout will stain and collect grunge. I worked for a maid service one summer while in college. One of my clients had just discovered the grout on her kitchen floor was dark from dirt and so my partner and I spent 2 hours on her kitchen floor cleaning grout, changing the black/grey grout back to white. I will never have a tile floor.

Other nonporous surfaces are Solid Surfacing, Quartz and Recycled Glass. So just remember that nonporous surfaces are easier to clean and do not require sealing. But just like cost, don't let that sway you from not getting a surface you have been dreaming of for years. Just know what to expect in maintenance.

Durability

There are certain hazards for a countertop that are inherit with being in the kitchen, they are: heat, knives, stains and water. Each countertop material has its own level of resistance for each of these. Many of the materials listed have great heat resistance and many also play well with water. However when it comes to knives, never use them directly on any countertop as the counter will suffer from direct contact with a knife blade. That being said, some materials are harder to scratch and some countertops can even have light scratches buffed out.

On the next page, I have put together a table listing the popular countertop materials and how well they hold up to scratches and scrapes. They are rated as follows:

1 Very Resistant

2 Somewhat Resistant

3 Be Careful

	Heat	Knives	Stains	Water
Laminates	3	2	2	1
Tile	1	1	1	1
Butcher Block	3	3	3	3
Granite	1	1	2	1
Solid Surface	3	3	2	1
Recycled Glass	1	1	1	1
Quartz	1	1	1	1
Marble	1	3	3	2
Stainless Steel	1	3	1	1
Soapstone	1	3	1	1
Concrete	1	2	2	2
Paper Composite	2	3	2	2

Colors

We have talked about materials from their practical side, what about colors? Sometimes the color you choose can also have a practical application. I have found that the speckled and spackled colors will hide crumbs very well. Depending on the kind of house keeper you are you may want the spackled color because no one will notice the crumbs on the counter unless they get down to eye level with the counter. But if you have a passion for cleanliness the spackled colors may not be for you because the crumbs are not easily seen and so easily missed.

Most all of these counter top materials come in a mindboggling selection of colors. Of course Butcher Block is wood color but you still have a wide range of brown coloring to choose from: light poplar all the way to a dark walnut. Concrete can even be stained to get the color you wish. Even soapstone which is traditionally black can now be obtained in a beautiful white with black streaks running through it. The White Soapstone I saw recently in a stone yard came from Italy. Don't let the color be your first guide in choosing a material.

Edges

When choosing a countertop, the salesman is going to ask you about the edge profile. The style of your kitchen will usually have a say in the edge of the counter top. If the kitchen is a sleek, clean cut, modern style the edge will be an Eased or Beveled profile. But if the kitchen is more ornate with decorative columns and large crown molding then an Ogee or Cove may be the answer. Google "countertop edge options" and all kinds of pictures will come up showing the options available.

Some products come with more edge options than others. The newer items such as the Paper Composite and concrete counter tops that are poured in place will often have limited choices. But I must mention that the straight sided profile are not totally flat as they will all have an eased or slightly rounded edge on the top and bottom. The edge is subject to knocks and bumps that can cause chips. Also the edge of stone and manufactured products can be very sharp. A slight rounding of that sharp edge will make the counter safe to use and keep the edge from chipping too easily.

Another word about concrete counter tops: They don't have to have a straight profile, there are forms that can be used to produce a different profile and that profile can be poured in place right with the countertop pour.

The old favorite, laminates, has had an explosion of edge options. The old style with the straight sides and exposed laminate edges is still available. The next option for laminates that was popular in the '90 was the use of a piece of stained oak trim to dress the edge. That really did look nice but now laminates have all kinds of edge profiles available and you no longer have to see the raw cut laminate edge.

There is something that is standard for all counter top materials; the more elaborate the profile, the more it will cost. Often the Eased (or Bevel) and Bullnose styles will come standard with the counter top. Here are examples of some standard edges.

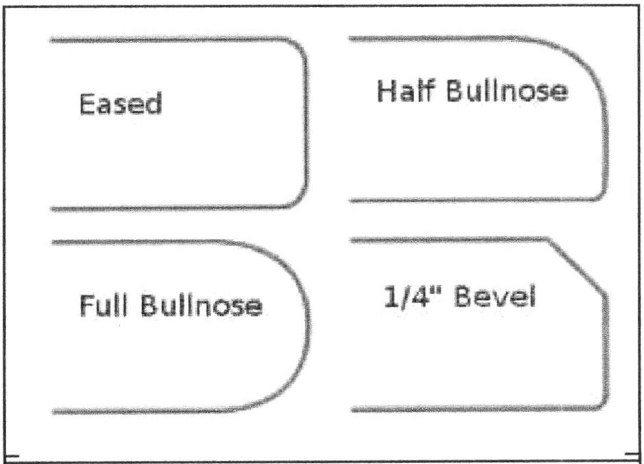

Countertop Edging

Sinks

There are two basic ways to mount a sink: drop-in or under mount. The sink itself may have a definite mount required but some are mountable either way. A drop-in sink is installed from the top and gets its name by dropping the sink (gently) into the countertop cut out. The sink is sealed around the edges to keep moisture from getting between the sink and the counter top and finding its way into the cabinet below. The under mount sink is installed from below and held up with clips fastened to the underside of the counter top which pinches the flange of the sink against the opening. The advantage to the under mount is that the crumbs from the counters are easily wiped into the sink whereas the rim on the drop-in sink gets in the way and can be harder to clean.

All counter tops can accommodate a drop-in sink, but not all can handle an under mount sink. The edge of the counter top is exposed with an under mount sink, so counters made from a laminate or even wood will not do well in this application.

A third type of sink that has become popular is the Farmhouse or Apron-Front sink. This sink has the front vertical surface of the sink showing. The Farmhouse sink is totally different from the other two. It is not supported by the counter top at all but by the cabinet itself. These sinks can get pretty heavy, up to 300 pounds when filled with water so extra supports must be added to the cabinet it will be mounted in. Also the cabinet front has to be modified to accommodate this type of sink.

A sink may also be integrated with a solid surface counter top in which case it is neither a drop-in or under mount but if it ever needs replacing, the whole counter top must be replaced. The advantage of an integrated sink is the elimination of any seams and therefore no caulking is required.

The sink itself can be made from different materials. Just looking at one of the box stores web sites I can see stainless steel, copper, granite, cast iron, fireclay, composite porcelain and acrylic sinks!

Copper sinks can be pricy but it is a very durable metal that will not rust and also has antimicrobial properties. Copper will change color over time but the patina that occurs is often considered desirable.

A granite sink is not actually a sink carved out of granite but a manmade item created from granite and acrylic that is sprayed over a resin base. This sink is very heat, stain and scratch resistant.

Cast iron is an old mainstay. Most homes from the 60s and 70s had cast iron sinks. These are heavy, durable sinks. They have a sound deadening quality that is not found in the stainless steel sinks. This sink is even more heat resistant than the granite sinks. It is the porcelain enamel finish that covers the cast iron that gives the sink its great attributes. There are many color options available for this great classic.

Porcelain sinks are often confused with the cast iron as they both have a porcelain enamel coating but the porcelain sink uses lighter gauge steel for the base metal. Like the cast iron it has superb heat resistance and is stain and scratch resistance. But one difference is noise; make sure the back is insulated to help deaden the sound.

The fireclay sink is heated to a high temperature when created to provide a durable sink that is chip and scratch resistant. These sinks come in a number of colors that will not fade or discolor. Being a non-porous surface it is bacteria resistant.

Composite sinks are created from a mixture of quartz or granite particles that are combined with an acrylic or polyester resin. This material is very hard and creates a very stain, scratch and chip resistant surface. Like the cast iron sink, this material has superb sound-deadening properties.

An acrylic sink is molded into the desired shape and reinforced with fiberglass or a composite to provide support and help deaden the sound. This material is stain resistant and handles impacts fairly well. This sink does scratch but they can often be polished out.

More commonly the sink is either porcelain enamel on cast iron or stainless steel. The more durable of the two is the stainless steel. If you choose to get a stainless steel sink, make sure it has sound proofing material applied to the underside. Even water running into the sink can sound loud without some sort of sound proofing on the sink.

A word of caution: stainless steel comes in various gauges (thickness). The gauge readings are rather counterintuitive. The bigger the gauge number, the <u>thinner</u> the steel. I highly recommend that nothing bigger than 18 gauge stainless be used. The 18 gauge will hold up better than the thinner 20 gauge sinks (think about dropping a dinner knife in the sink, or the sink supporting a garbage disposal). I know this sounds backwards, but the smaller the gauge number, the thicker the metal. Sinks can also be found in 16 gauge which is thicker than 18 but will be more expensive. Another issue with the thinner metal is that they make the faucet feel cheap because the sink will give and flex every time the water is turned on and the sink will be more prone to dents. So just don't get anything thinner than an 18 gauge sink.

Choose a corrosion resistant stainless. Let me get technical for a minute. The 300 series stainless has a high amount of chromium and nickel which improves the corrosion resistance; 304 and 316 series are considered the best. If you can stick a magnet to the inside of the sink, it is made from a lower-quality stainless and should be avoided.

Sinks will also vary by the number of basins or bowls. A single basin makes it easy to clean large pots and pans or small children. Double sinks give you a bowl for soapy water and a second bowl for rinse water. Double sinks also allow a person to rinse fruits and vegetables in one side while stacking the dirties in the other as they cook. Triple bowl sinks are also available. There are many options for sizes but which ever sink you choose most will fit easily in a 36 inch sink base cabinet. Smaller sinks can be found that will fit in a 33 inch sink base. The farmhouse or apron sink will require a special sink base.

The two bowls do not have to be the same size. Sometimes it is helpful to have a larger bowl and then a smaller shallower bowl for washing vegetables. One bowl may be inset from the wall to allow room for the faucet behind it or the two bowls may look the same just that one is narrower with the faucet behind the two bowls. Common proportions for the two bowl sink are 50/50, 60/40 and 70/30.

Another consideration about the sink is depth. Most people like the idea of a really deep sink but it can get too deep. The standard kitchen sink depth is 8 inches deep but they can very anywhere from 6 inches to 10 inches. The shallower basins feel cheap and just don't hold much of anything. But the deep sinks have their own problems.

If you desire a really deep sink, under-mount a deep sink, that will provide another inch or two to the depth. Just remember that the deeper the sink the farther down you will have to reach to get to the bottom of the sink. Some people do not like leaning over the sink to work in it.

I lived in a house once that had a deep 9 ½ inch sink that was under mounted in a quartz countertop that was 1 ½ inch thick so that sink was 11 inches deep! This deep of a sink meant I had to lean over to get to the bottom of the sink. So remember if the sink is under mounted, that will add to the depth of the sink.

If you are looking for more volume in the sink, changing the shape may do it for you. Square corners with straight sides and flat bottoms will hold more water than the rounded corners of most sinks. However, the rounded corners will make the sink easier to clean, getting into those tight corners can be difficult.

And finally make sure your sink will handle the accessories you may want. The faucet may require one hole or three. There are other items that may be desired at the sink such as separate spray head, built in soap dispenser or even a dedicated hot water tap.

It is amazing the variety of sinks available and also bewildering. Not only is there a variety of sinks but also a variety of faucets! Spend a little more money and get a very good faucet. A cheap faucet will be a bother to you as long as you have it.

Countertop installation

This should be a short section. Don't do this yourself. Most counter tops should be installed by a professional. Many places that sell the stone and manmade composite countertops will also handle the installation. Often installation is included in the price of the stone. These businesses know this is an expensive item and they want it installed right. What usually happens is that after the cabinets are installed, the counter top installers will show up, often with some fancy computerized measuring tools, and will take measurements. They realize that walls are seldom plumb or square so these measurements take this into consideration. They then go back to the shop and layout the measurements and cut the stone or other material. The counter may actually be in two or three or more pieces. When they come back in a couple of days they will install the countertop and with more special equipment they will draw the pieces tight together with an adhesive sealant between them.

For the home owner with construction skills, installation of wooden or even a laminate counter top is possible, if you are adventurous. Just take careful measurements and remember that walls are seldom square or plumb and make allowances. By becoming knowledgeable about the techniques, concrete counters may also be within the skill set of some home owners.

Special uses

The first uses that come to mind are pastry making and bread making. Many people may consider these to require the same type of counter top. The same lower 30" cabinet height is useful for both, but actually they are two different events that like different surfaces.

Let's start with pastry. This can be for cookies or pie crust but the actions are pretty much the same. Pastry making involves mixing dough in a bowl, with or without a mixer, and then rolling the dough out on a surface. For pastry, the surface needs to be cool, that helps the dough release from the surface. A cool surface also helps keep the solid fats from melting, which affects the texture of the dough. A cool surface is also required for laminating doughs and quickly cooling pastry cream. Most stones are high mass, dense surfaces and so usually provide the cool that is required. Marble is a traditional stone used for pastries. Be aware that marble is a soft stone and if it is not cleaned soon after use it can absorb the oils in the dough which can discolor the stone. Some people enjoy the patina as it shows use. Granite is another stone but I would be leery of this one because it is porous and the little holes and crevices will collect dough if not property sealed. A better option to granite may be quartz for this application. The same type of surface that works well for pastry also works well for candy making that requires a cool surface.

The second activity is bread making. Unlike pastry, breads prefer a warm counter. Many people really prefer wood for this. This wood can be a section of butcher block or could be a large wood cutting board that is only brought out when needed. The wood helps spread the flour more evenly under the dough which makes for a higher quality product. If you are really into bread making, the expense of a heated countertop may be worthwhile. These heating mats can be installed under a countertop just like radiant heating is installed under floors.

Another interesting use for a countertop is not actually a countertop. Use some of your beautiful stone counter material as an accent by running it down the end of the cabinet like a waterfall. This produces a flow effect where your eye is drawn across the top and down the side following the counter to the floor. This can look very dramatic. You may even choose to use a different material for this accent surface to make it even more dramatic. The next picture shows this effect on an island.

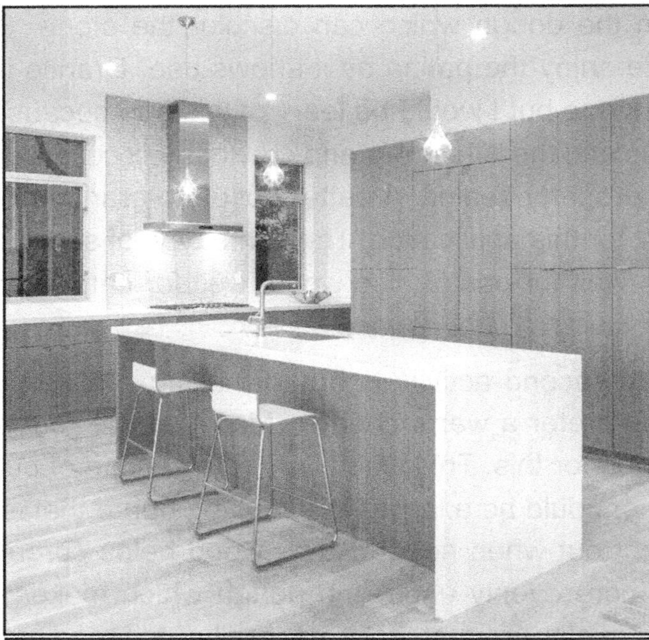

Countertop Waterfall Example
Photo by BondRocketImages/Shutterstock

But let us get back to function.

Food preparation area

The best location for the hard working food prep area is between the sink and the stove or cooktop. If the stove and sink are not connected by a continuous counter top, such as the sink is on an island, choose a section of counter top by the sink as first choice and by the stove as second choice. The space needs to be at least 36 inches long with 42 inches being desirable. If the space gets to be too long the functionality is actually decreased. Too many steps to get from the stove to the sink are inefficient. However, if 48 inches are available for this workspace, go for it.

Reserve this space for food prep. Try not to store other things such as coffee pots, toasters, microwaves in this area. The full depth (usually 24-25 inches) is needed for cutting board, ingredients, cookbook and other tools actually in use for meal preparation.

If the food preparation area makes a 90 degree turn at a corner, count the total linear feet down the front of the countertop. For example; if you have two feet of space at the front of the counter between the sink and the corner and then another two feet between the corner and the stove, this gives the 4 feet or 48 inches for the work area.

Some kitchens have two or more work areas. When planning for more than one cook, consider where each will be and what they may be doing. Remember that the sink is the hardest working area in the kitchen. Two cooks will need to have access to the sink from their work station. If the second work station is more than a step from the sink (meaning 4 feet) consider adding another sink. Someone making a salad will need access to the refrigerator, sink and preparation area. Someone heating vegetables in the microwave will need access to wherever the vegetables are stored, the sink to wash the vegetables, a work surface and the microwave. Someone using the oven will need access to a work surface, and the oven. Just consider the possibilities and plan for them.

For more information and to see the above picture in color, go to https://akitchenyoulove.com/ch4

Chapter 5
Backsplashes

"Discoveries are often made by not following instructions, by going off the main road, by trying the untried."
—Frank Tyger

Purpose of backsplash

The backsplash is to protect the exposed wall behind the countertop with an easy to clean surface. The wall between the counter top and wall cabinet is notorious for being splashed with food and liquids. The sink area gets water splashes and the stove area gets grease splashes and everything in between gets all manner of splashes (maybe that is why it is called a back 'splash')

A painted wall offers some protection, but the texturing – even if just texturing from the paint – has crevices that will try and hold any particles that get on it. Scrubbing the wall may rub off the paint, creating more problems. Therefore most people opt to put in a backsplash.

Short or full

The first question to ask is, will the backsplash be short or will you go for full coverage? Most people like the look of a backsplash that goes all the way to the bottom of the wall cabinets. Such a backsplash will protect the wall well and when it comes to cleaning, you don't have to worry about getting cleaner on the painted wall.

But there may be times when a shorter backsplash may be desired. It is much easier to hang items on the wall when you don't have to drill through tile or some other hard material. A shorter backsplash may make electrical boxes and their cover plates easier to deal with. Some prefabricated countertop materials come with a short 4 inch backsplash installed free of charge. And then there is money, less here means more to spend elsewhere.

A short backsplash does not necessarily mean 4 inches. Look at the picture of the kitchen with all the plugs in the electrical chapter to come. Just below that electrical plug strip is a glass backsplash. Above the strip is just painted wall. The backsplash is encased between the countertop and the electrical plug strip. This is tall enough to catch all but the most exuberant splashes.

Now let's look at some common backsplash materials.

Tile

This is probably the most used backsplash material. It is versatile, comes in any number of colors, sizes and shapes and has a wide price range. I like tile. It is easy to clean and is impervious to water, however grout is not.

The one thing I do not like about tile is the grout. Grout holds stains. What about that red wine that gets splashed on the tile? The memory will linger in the grout line. The staining problem may be reduced by tightening the spacing between tiles and by being picky about the grout used. I have used an unsanded grout that was almost like rubber when it dried. This grout cleaned just as easily as the tile! The only drawback with that rubbery grout was with installation. I had to be very careful and tape all the edges where I did not want this compound because it would stick and not come off.

Tile is also great for creating a focal point. Such areas are usually behind the range where a taller expanse of wall is available. If there is no kitchen window, the illusion of a window can be created with a focal point of tile above the sink. Using a different tile or even the same tile but in a different pattern for the focal point can be very pleasing to the eye.

Tile can become dated quickly. If you want a classic kitchen that will withstand the fickle nature of fashion, choose a white tile in a simple pattern such as subway tile or some other rectangular shape. Of course if you are creating a kitchen to go with a time period, choose something that fits that time frame. Then again if you see something you just fall in love with, use that. If you get tired of it in a few years, it can be changed out without a major expense.

Paint

Ok, I kind of negated the idea of a painted backsplash earlier but I wanted to mention it as a possibility. It is very versatile, more so than tile. The paint can always be a solid color and that color could be changed out as often as you are willing to bring out the paint cans. But there is another side to painting a backsplash that really brings out your creative side.

How about Faux painting? Just look up painted backsplash ideas on www.pinterest.com and you will see all kinds of faux painting. Some look simple enough for a novice. And if you have an artistic streak, this could be your canvas.

The wallboard, textured or not, does not have to be the canvas. How about painting beadboard, or the metal or faux metal ceiling tiles and attaching them to the wall. With the proper paint, you can even paint the back of plate glass. Don't like your existing tile backsplash? That could be painted too. So don't let me dissuade you from paint as a backsplash, just be aware of its limitations.

Glass

I mentioned glass above. Now I am not talking glass tiles which are small pieces that come in 12 inch by 12 inch sheets at $30 per sheet and have grout lines. I am talking about a solid sheet of glass that stretches from one wall to the other. This can look very contemporary, think IKEA loft. It has very clean lines and will not work in a frilly kitchen. This type of backsplash is very easy to clean, just spray it with window cleaner and wipe down.

As a kitchen designer, I am going to tell you to use tempered glass. But I know, if I leave you to your own devices, you won't. Simple plate glass is so much cheaper than tempered and tempered glass has to have all outlet holes precut before tempering as the glass cannot be cut afterwards. So if you must, use ¼ inch thick or more glass. Don't even consider using this un-tempered glass if someone in the home is rough in the kitchen.

Regular plate glass has a green cast to it so test any wall color behind the glass before deciding on the wall color. Glass can be obtained that is more optically clear but it is very expensive. Also as mentioned above, the back of the glass can be painted. It will require special paint to keep it from peeling later. It will also be good to space the glass out from the wall slightly so the painted wall does not stick to the glass (or painted glass does not stick to the wall). There are spacers that can be used for this that look sharp and contemporary.

If the glass is not painted, get it lightly sandblasted. This will help hide the imperfections in the wall behind. In fact if the wall behind has been heavily textured, get a medium to heavy sandblasting on your glass. Again, get samples and hold them up to your wall and see which hides it the best. All little ripples and imperfections in the wall will be seen through the glass.

I have also seen some very beautiful fused glass backsplashes. These were works of art and priced as such.

Metal

Another unusual material to use is stainless steel. As a sheet product, stainless can be shiny which is what one thinks of when thinking of a professional kitchen. This will make the kitchen look very serious and clean. But stainless can also be brushed which will dull the shine considerably. Or have some fun and distress your own using all manner of devices. This will make the kitchen look more youthful, vibrant and contemporary.

Then there are metal tiles. These come in various shapes, sheens and sizes. The metal tiles often have a ceramic backing and are set just like ceramic or porcelain wall tiles. Use a non-sanded grout to prevent scratching the metal. You will also want to use a metal edge piece to finish the tile to the surrounding wall at any exposed edges.

This metal is not limited to stainless steel. Tiles and sheet are also found in aluminum and copper and for tiles, sometimes a mixture of these.

Countertop as backsplash

Some people like the look of continuity with the countertop material running right up the wall. Maybe just running it up the critical 4 inches is plenty for you. The wall above that can be painted or finished with some other treatment.

There is no law that says the countertop material used has to be what is on the counter. Try a solid piece of marble or soapstone for the backsplash. Both of those are soft stones and are not recommended for extensive countertop use but as a backsplash that gets little wear, it should do fine. Butcher block is also a potential backsplash material.

Wallpaper

This could be one of the cheapest and most elaborate looks but I really don't recommend it except as a temporary backsplash. This will not hold up well to repeated scrubbing or dampness. Use one of the vinyl wallpapers if you must throw something up on the wall to protect it while you wait for your more permanent material to come in. Using a finishing strip, such as a painted or stained quarter-round, will cover the edges nicely and also keep them from curling up if they come loose. If you happen to really like your wallpaper backsplash consider putting a layer of clear glass over it. The glass will protect the paper and is also super easy to clean.

Something almost like wallpaper is self-adhesive tile sheets. These are easier to apply than the wallpaper and can quickly transform a space. But here again I would only consider this as temporary. These come in a large array of patterns and colors and if you are stymied about what to do with your backsplash, buy several patterns of self-adhesive tiles and try them out one at a time and see which pattern appeals to you. For a little money and little effort you can be confident in your pattern and color choice and purchase the more expensive real thing. Some of these tiles seem to be stickier than others so you may want to stick them to a thin sheet of plywood tacked against the wall that way it will be easier to remove and change out later. If that is going to be your permanent backsplash go ahead and stick it to the wall.

Be creative

This is an opportunity to express yourself. Take a walk through your local builder supply store and look at all the different materials there as potential backsplash material. Like a wood look tile? Put it on the wall. Don't just consider finish materials, there are various building materials that may work also. The building supply section is where you can find sheets of metal, but you may need to go to a tile store to get the metal trim to finish the edge.

Flooring material can also be used on the wall. In the early 1900's, linoleum flooring was used as a cheap countertop material so why not use other flooring for the backsplash.

Also consider other wall materials for use as a non-traditional backsplash. People have used shiplap and beadboard for the backsplash for a great look. Other nontraditional materials include pallet wood which needs to be sanded down to keep the splinter potential down. But pallet wood can be stained, even staining individual pieces in different colors for a real rustic look.

To really let your creativity run wild consider breaking plates, cups and tiles and creating your own mosaic backsplash. Any number of items can be imbedded in the mortar including old pieces of silverware and even jewelry pieces.

Another interesting backsplash is slices of fossilized rock. This is often sandstone or limestone which is rather porous and would benefit being behind glass.

The backsplash can be the masterpiece of your kitchen. My parting advice on the backsplash is to make it yours but also make it match the style and look of your kitchen. The backsplash does not stand alone.

Check out some amazing backspash ideas at https://akitchenyoulove.com/ch5

Chapter 6
What's Underfoot

> *"It is not the beauty of a building you should look at; it's the construction of the foundation that will stand the test of time."*
> *—David Allan Coe*

Flooring

This section is almost like the section on countertops, there are so many choices and new choices seem to be added every year. Some materials go in and out of style, so if you are redesigning for your own use and not just to resell in the next year or two, go with the material you really want. If you are planning on reselling in five years, what you choose now may be considered out of date and worn out by then so I emphasize again, just get what works for you at this time.

Tile

Tile has been a popular choice of floor covering for kitchens and bathrooms for a long time. A classic choice in tile can maintain its popularity for many years but the wrong choice can really date the space. Tiles may either be ceramic or porcelain. If at all possible, choose porcelain. The porcelain is a tougher material less susceptible to chips and cracks. Also the color runs deeper in porcelain than in ceramic tile so if it does chip it may not be as noticeable.

Tile can be slippery when wet so be sure to get a tile rated for floors. The grout lines help make a tile less slippery and that is one reason why small tiles are used in shower floors. Consider matching the grout to the tile. Grout can be dyed to any number of colors. A colored grout may also hide the dirt that always seems to collect in the grout joints.

Wood

Wood is also a popular flooring choice, especially when one wants the kitchen floor to flow easily into the family or dining room. One floor can cover all three areas. There are a number of ways to finish wood floors. Discuss with your floor finisher about what is the best finish for a wood floor to be used in the kitchen. But even with the most resilient finish, get the spills off the floor as soon as possible as wood is susceptible to water damage.

Laminate

Laminate flooring can give you the look of wood but without the cost. Laminates come in all types of wood color from the ash grays through the dark walnuts and even exotic woods like zebra wood and tiger wood. Not only can you get wood look a-likes but also laminate that looks like tile, stone and even metal.

This is a versatile product and easy for a do-it-yourselfer to install. This product has been around for quite a while and the more recent laminates have increased their quality but I am still leery about using them in the kitchen.

Laminates are made by gluing a high-resolution image of real wood to a core of fiberboard. This fiberboard is backed by a treated bottom layer that is supposed to prevent moisture damage. This whole board is then covered by a clear wear layer to help resist scuffs and scratches. However even with the treated bottom layer and the clear coat application, laminates are still susceptible to water damage. If you are fast at cleaning up spills and splashes this floor may work for you. I know it would not work for me; my refrigerator has been known to spit out an ice cube with no one around and let it melt on the floor. Laminates also have a characteristic hollow sound with hard soled and high heeled shoes. Many people do not care for that sound.

There is a hybrid product that combines the benefits of laminates but has a real wood veneer so that it can take an occasional refinishing – but that depends on the thickness of the veneer.

Sheet vinyl

This product has been used for years and is still a staple for wet or dirty environments such as laundries, mud rooms, entry ways, bathrooms, utility rooms, and kitchens. Vinyl is popular due to its lower cost, ability to withstand moisture and ease of cleaning. Although large rolls of vinyl can be purchased at your local large box store, I would not recommend the average home owner attempt installation themselves. One slip of the utility knife and you have an unintentional seam. Leave the installation to professionals who do it every day – they are artists!

Vinyl comes in 12, 13.2, and even 15.5 foot wide sheets. If the room is larger than this, there will be an intentional seam.

There are many styles to choose from. Whether it is tile, wood, stone, concrete or even a metal look, you can find it in vinyl. The higher quality vinyl will have the more realistic look.

Vinyl does have its problems: it can be torn and heavy objects can leave an imprint. I have seen refrigerators leave dents and ranges leave gouges on a vinyl floor. Here again the better quality flooring will hold up better to such abuse.

Vinyl also comes in peel and stick squares. This can be useful in the rental housing market. When one tile gets damaged the tile can be removed and another one laid down. However for every day, long term use I do not recommend it. I have seen too many tiles with curled edges and some that seem to lose their stick ability. Also with the individual tiles one of the main functions of the flooring is lost, that of being impervious to water. All those seams between the tiles will let moisture in.

Linoleum

That is a term that was not used for many years but it has now resurfaced (ha, ha). Linoleum is considered to be very durable - warranties can range as high as 25 years. It's also eco-friendly; that is why there is heightened interest in it today. The flooring has a nice resiliency to it that makes it nice to walk on. Vinyl and cork are also resilient floors. Resiliency is a desirable quality in a kitchen where a cook may be standing and walking for an hour while preparing a meal. Yes, contrary to popular belief, people do still cook.

Linoleum is made from linseed oil, pine resins, wood flour and cork powder. It is the cork which gives it the bounce. Linoleum takes dye very well and can be found in a rainbow of colors – and also many more subtle colors. This color runs throughout the material not just on the surface as with vinyl and laminates.

The flooring is susceptible to scratches and fading from sunlight exposure. But with the color being throughout the linoleum, scratches are not as easily seen. Some manufacturers add a coating to their linoleum which will help protect the flooring from scratching and sunlight. If no coating is available, the flooring really should be cleaned and waxed every two to three year to help it keep its luster. With proper care this floor could last 40 years or better. An interesting contradiction is that even though it has a long useful life, it is biodegradable which is another plus for the ecologically minded.

Linoleum sounds like the perfect flooring but it does have its problems. High heels and furniture legs can dent it. Sharp objects can cut it. As mentioned above, sunlight can darken or yellow the flooring – if not protected. And the biggie is that linoleum can be susceptible to moisture and so is not recommended for use in bathrooms, laundry rooms or in the kitchen if you are not diligent about wiping up spills and splashes.

After installation a smell is emitted but it is not harmful VOCs but just the odor from the linseed oil and that will disappear after a couple of weeks.

This product is manufactured as glue-down sheets which I recommend a professional install. But it also comes as snap-together tiles that will satisfy the do-it-yourselfer.

Other floor products

There are a couple more floors I wanted to bring up: Concrete and Vinyl plank.

Concrete floors are a versatile alternative. They are easy to install especially when building a new house. The concrete can be dyed to any number of colors; it can also be scored to make it look like large tile blocks. A wax and buff process finishes the look. This is one of the more economical floors if installed with the initial build. It is also a floor I think is best left to a professional.

The main drawback for a concrete floor is that it is hard on the feet. If you don't actually spend much time in the kitchen this may be ok. A soft mat can also be used at the sink and the prep area to help out the feet and back. Another note drawn on the surface hardness is that things dropped on it may easily break.

Any chips in the concrete may be buffed down but there will still be a divot. The color is mixed in the original concrete so it will show true with any ding. If a divot is large you may be tempted to patch it. Just be aware it may be difficult to match the color exactly.

Another product I really like for a number of reasons is vinyl plank flooring. This material is made completely out of vinyl with fiberglass reinforcement! This means it is totally impervious to water! Which makes it great flooring for the bath, laundry or kitchen. You can soak a piece in water for a week and it will not absorb any of it. There are actually two versions of this floor. One is a snap-together product and the other is a glue-down version. I am only considering the snap-together version in this section. The glue down is messy to apply and then to remove later, it can also gap and buckle when the floor it is glued to expands and contracts due to humidity or temperature. The snap-together version floats between the walls so does not have this problem.

Another notable advantage of the vinyl plank is that it has a resiliency that makes it easy to walk on. I love the feel underfoot. Even the thinner, lower priced products from the big box stores feel good. This resiliency will also provide some give if a plate is dropped on it and the item may actually survive the fall where as if the floor was tile or concrete the item might break.

The vinyl plank is also a great project for the do-it-yourselfer. These planks click together like laminate floor, but they cut easier than the laminate. All that is required is a utility knife with a sharp blade. You will need to replace the blades fairly frequently because the fiberglass in the vinyl plank wears the blades out quickly. The plank is scored and then bent to snap the score – kind of like scoring and snapping drywall. A pair of tin-snips can be used for more complex cuts, but the cut will tend to be more ragged so this only works where the edge will be covered up with something else like an escutcheon plate or a vent register.

This product also comes in a wide price range. I have found many of the cheaper product performs as well or sometimes better than the more expensive versions. I have used an economical product from Lowes and special ordered a more expensive product from a local flooring store and I must say the more expensive product kept coming unclicked while installing the floor. So my advice is that before you buy, snap a couple of mating samples together and make sure they grip well.

Although the vinyl plank is impervious to water, I still like to put a waterproof membrane under it to protect the subfloor from any water that may seep through the cracks of the planks. Another down side is that the plank may take a set from heavy objects.

Cost

Each of these floorings comes in a range of prices. Usually you get what you pay for (however see the section about vinyl plank). Part of the cost involved will be installation. If you are on a tight budget and want to do-it-yourself your choices may be limited to what you are willing to tackle.

The more expensive versions of a product will usually be able to handle abuse better and stay nice looking for a longer time. If you like the idea of changing things out every few years, (or having an excuse to change things out) go with the cheaper versions.

Flooring is usually priced out on a cost per square foot basis. This makes it easier to compare products. However you will not be able to buy the products by the square foot. Concrete is usually sold by the yard when using a cement mixer or by the bag when mixed by hand. Sheet linoleum and sheet vinyl is sold by the foot in length and the rolls come in specific widths. Wood flooring like laminates and the vinyl plank comes in boxes of varying coverage amounts. Tile comes in boxes of a certain count and sometimes individually. The tile sizes themselves will vary in their size and so in their coverage. Take good measurements of your space and calculate how much flooring you need, then look at the increments your flooring comes in. If your room is 11 feet wide and 10 feet long and the sheet linoleum comes in 12 foot widths, you will need at least a 10 foot length of the flooring. But always add an extra 10% to the amount, as there will be mistakes and oops and unsquared rooms.

Maintenance and durability

I have touched on the durability of each product while talking about each above. There are some things to consider when deciding on a floor from the durability stand point.

The main consideration is your lifestyle. Are you fastidious in your house cleaning? Personally I have better things to do with my time than clean. So I gravitate toward items that are easy to clean or better yet hide dirt. Now you know my dirty secret. If spills are left on the floor for more than 10 minutes choose one of the floors that can handle that such as Vinyl plank or sheet, Tile, or Concrete.

Another area to consider is do you have pets that would be hard on a floor? A large dog may have claws that can scratch some surfaces. I lived in a house once that had a large Terrazzo entry and when we bought the house, the surface next to the wall was all scratched where over the years the dog had run to the door. I was able to take most of the scratches out by stripping, waxing and buffing the floor. I currently have cats, so the only issue I have is keeping the furball tumbleweeds at bay. Floors that are good with scratches include Concrete, Tile, and some Woods or Laminates. It may surprise you that I said tile when I just told you my experience with the Terrazzo. Certain stones such as Marble and some man-made tiles like Terrazzo are considered soft and have to be treated and cleaned with special cleaners; they cannot tolerate harsh chemicals usually used to clean hard surface floors.

Another consideration is how often you actually use the kitchen for extensive lengths of time. Are you an occasional cook? Only cooking on special occasions? Do you mainly reheat frozen foods or do you enjoy preparing home cooked meals several times a week? This will tell you if you need a resilient floor such as Vinyl plank or sheet, Linoleum, Wood, or Laminates. These are softer and easier to stand on for long periods of time. I am an avid cook and will often spend 1-2 hours at a time in the kitchen preparing foods several times a week so I want a resilient floor. Of course you can always buy soft mats to place at critical areas such as the sink, the stove and the preperation area. I am always looking at maintenance and having to take care of added mats does not fit my style, but maybe it would work for you.

From the above information, the flooring that fits me and my style would be Vinyl Plank or Sheet Vinyl. But that fits me not you. Each person has their own needs, wants and biases and a good kitchen designer will suggest a flooring material to fit those desires.

Maintenance

Each floor has different methods of cleaning and maintaining. Please follow the guidelines of the manufacture. Read product labels to see if they will work for you. Tile is probably the easiest and most forgiving on cleaning methods and chemicals. The top wax used on concrete, woods and linoleums may limit your cleaning methods and tools. For my impervious floors I have a Hoover Floormate (because I hate mopping) but when it finally dies I think I will get a steam cleaner as I have a friend who just swears by hers. But I would never use that on Laminates or a Wood floor. Follow the manufacturer's recommendations and your floor will stay nice, clean and in good shape for years to come.

Style of home

One last thought, consider the flavor of your home. Does it have a Spanish or Moorish influence? Then tile might fit in better than the other products. Is it Mid-Century Modern? Going with Linoleum would be a safe choice. A Wood floor would be at home in a Cape Cod.

So take style into consideration but if you really want Wood in your Spanish ranch, be eclectic and do what you really want. There is no rule that you have to be authentic to the style. But if you are at a loss as to what type of floor to put in, ask the house, it may tell you.

See pictures at https:akitchenyoulove.com/ch6

Chapter 7
Elephants In The Room

"Ideas are like rabbits. You get a couple and learn how to handle them, and pretty soon you have a dozen."
—John Steinbeck

Basics

Most people know what appliances go into a kitchen: Refrigerator/Freezer, Stove or range top and wall ovens, and more often than not, a dishwasher. The microwave is becoming such a basic appliance in the kitchen that its location needs to be considered in the planning stage as well. Many of these appliances come in various sizes and shapes, especially the refrigerator. Dealing with the large items can feel like managing elephants.

Size

Be careful when purchasing a refrigerator, make sure it will fit in the space planned. Most full size refrigerators will fit in a 36 inch wide opening but there are some that are wider. Often people forget to check the height. Refrigerators can vary a lot in height and if cabinets are installed above the appliance there could be a conflict. Remember to include the top of the hinge in the height measurement. Refrigerators also come in different depths. The 'counter depth' refrigerator is becoming more popular but even these are not standardized in their depth. If you really want one that does not stick out past the counter (which is usually 25 inches) be sure and check measurements. Be aware that for the door to open past 90 degrees - so drawers will actually slide out - the refrigerator may have to stick out from the edge of the counter slightly. For this reason, do not and I repeat, *do not* install a refrigerator against a side wall which keeps the refrigerator door from opening wide enough for the drawers to slide out.

The dishwasher is more standardized in its size. A 24 inch hole is needed for the dishwasher and if it is installed at the end of a cabinet run, an end panel will be needed to hide the side of the dishwasher and supply support for the countertop. The dishwasher should not be mounted more than 36 inches from the sink. The dishwasher usually taps into the sink's water supply and drain. Be sure to run any flooring into the dishwasher's slot, this will allow the dishwasher to sit properly and allow you or a repairman to actually slide it out if needed.

A stand-alone stove or range –the kind you see at the appliance stores all siting in a row with finished sides – is traditionally 30 inches wide. This will be covered in more detail a little farther on in this chapter, as will each of the basic appliances.

Frills

There are a number of appliances that many people would consider as a 'like to have' but not a necessity except for those people that have them, they have become a necessity. Years ago, the dishwasher was considered an extravagant frill and you were somebody if you had one. The microwave is a similar item. Nowadays almost every kitchen has a dishwasher and microwave.

How about an espresso machine? These can be obtained as countertop models for $40 or if you are willing to spend a somewhat larger amount (up to $4,000) a sleek built in model is available. It all depends on your taste and budget.

Something more likely to become a necessity is an under the counter ice maker, especially in hot climates. My husband can go through 5 pounds of ice on a hot summer day. Many refrigerators have ice makers with indoor dispensers but their capacity is limited and they eat into the freezer space.

On the other end of the spectrum are warming drawers. They are great if you are always hosting dinner parties.

How about a wine or beverage cooler? Many people think that is the ultimate must have. Taking the wine cooler a step farther; how about a multi-bottle wine dispenser. Just remember all of these items take up cabinet space which is often highly coveted in a small or even medium size kitchen.

Then there are items that can be very handy for those who frequently use such appliances. How about an in counter steamer/rice cooker? This could lend itself to healthier eating if actually used. A water source needs to be nearby. Continuing with water, what about a pot-filler at the cook top? The water would still have to be dumped out afterwards but if boiling water seems to be constantly on the stove, this may be a requirement for you. Just don't try to use this to put out a grease fire!

Appliance doors

A note about doors on appliances: they open. There should be plenty of passage way around an appliance when the door is open. Many appliances list their depth when the door is closed and when the door is open. This is found under specifications on the dealer's website.

When two appliances are across from each other there is potential need for both doors to be open at once and this can cause problems as both may be fighting for the same floor space.

Another potential problem is an inside corner. If the appliance is too close to the adjacent corner the knobs and handles on the doors and drawers can interfere with opening the appliance door! Of course the best solution is not put an appliance so close to a corner that you cannot stand between the open door and the adjacent cabinets. It is always best to be able to walk all the way around the front of an open appliance.

There is much more on this topic in the next chapter.

Hide and seek

There are ways to hide some appliances. Many cabinet manufacturers have panels that can be inserted into the front of dishwashers or attached to refrigerators. By making such a large item like the refrigerator look like part of the cabinetry, the space will feel less cluttered and the kitchen will have cleaner lines. This is purely a personal design and budget choice. The one appliance I have never seen hidden is the range.

The refrigerator could be hidden by taking it out of the big box. There are under the counter refrigerators available. These come in either a door style that swings like a mini version of a standard refrigerator or drawers that pull open and each drawer can be set to its own particular temperature.

Of course there are the popular appliance garages that keep bulky counter top appliances like toasters hidden away until needed. However, if the item is used daily it is best to just leave it in plain site as that is where it is likely to end up anyway. One of the problems with appliance garages is the door swing. Remember the section above on appliance doors, well this is just another version of that. Items will invariably end up sitting in front of the appliance garage. Some doors swing out like a walk door which means the items in front of it must be moved. Some doors have a top hinge where they swing up like some flat panel garage doors. These still need a clear space in front. There is even a version of this style that levers the door up keeping it parallel to the opening (not hinged at the top) but this version blocks the opening of any door of the cabinet above the garage. The door requiring the least amount of opening space is a roll top or tambour style (think of a roll top desk).

Let us tackle each appliance in turn.

Refrigerator

This is the main elephant in the room. It really sticks out, sometimes very literally. Some don't stick out as far as others, such as the counter depth refrigerators. There are many versions of the counter depth refrigerator. One is actually a commercial refrigerator. They look snazzy with their glass fronts. But be aware that they are not built like residential refrigerators. Commercial refrigerators are uninsulated and use far more energy than a residential refrigerator. The commercial version is also very difficult and expensive to repair. Some areas may even require a variance to place a commercial refrigerator in your home. However the commercial look (maybe not to the extent of glass see-through doors) can be had from stainless steel residential refrigerators.

Professional refrigerators are different from the commercial units but are actually designed to look like a commercial unit with the compressor on the top. Sub-Zero makes a refrigerator that is a close match as it has the compressor on top and a glass door option. These professional refrigerators are wider than the normal residential version. These are BIG appliances some are 52 inches wide, be sure to read the appliance information for sizing.

Then there are the Residential refrigerators. Even these have different versions. There is the standard slide it into a box opening in the cabinets; these may stick out 2 to 6 inches. Then there are those that are built into a housing where the sides will sit flush with the surrounding cabinets. The refrigerator still sticks out about 2 inches to allow door clearance. Then there is what is called "panel-ready" refrigerators. These will accept a panel that matches the rest of the kitchen cabinetry. This is sometimes called "Overlay" which is just the built-in version of the panel door. But even with this built-in version, the refrigerator will still protrude out into the kitchen some. To completely camouflage this behemoth it has to be integrated. This is the next type. On integrated refrigerators there are no compressor vents seen and they are built with an inset door that allows it to be in perfect alignment with the surrounding cabinets. This style will cause a guest to have to hunt for where the refrigerator is because it just does not look like one.

Let's go back to the standard refrigerators after that heady trek through the high end refrigerators. What can you get at your standard appliance store? A lot! There are all kinds of styles and colors and even widths. Style includes: Side-by-Side, French Door, Bottom Freezer, Top Freezer, Four-door and even Freezerless Refrigerators. Colors or surface can vary just as much. There is the standard black and white and now stainless steel has become standard. A popular color in recent years is slate with a new version popping up called Grey. I have also seen Bisque and I understand Avocado Green and Harvest Gold are making a comeback as a nod to the retro scene. About widths, always check the documentation on the refrigerator to make sure it will fit where you want it to go. It is embarrassing when you have a 36 inch space and the refrigerator shows up and it is 36.5 inches.

Don't forget compact refrigerators that can slide under the counter. These will include some of the specialty coolers such as beverage centers. By–the-way these can also come panel ready. The refrigerator drawer falls in the under the counter category. A compact refrigerator can also be taller than counter height and these will often contain a freezer with its own exterior door.

The number of options available is just wild. But remember, anything out of the ordinary ("off the shelf" from an appliance store) will cost more. Even the small compacts will be expensive if you figure cost per cubic foot of usable space.

Dishwashers

These are a lot less complicated than the refrigerators. There are three basic models; 18 inch built-in, 24 inch built-in, and the portable. If space is at a premium the smaller 18 inch version may be the answer. It can come panel ready and Energy Star Certified just like the 24 inch version which is more common. All three can be found with stainless steel interiors.

Colors for dishwashers are all over the place just like for the refrigerators; Black, White, Stainless Steel, Silver, Grey, Slate, Bisque and I have also seen Red. The controls can be on top of the door, so it hides when the door is closed, or on a front panel.

One thing that can vary a lot is the noise level. There are those that are as quiet as 38 dB (Decibel) and those that go over 60 dB. To give you an example 30 dB can sound like a whisper where 60 is conversational speech or an air conditioner, this is loud enough to make it hard to talk over. By most standards, 41 to 46 decibels is considered quiet. A note about sound – Decibels readings are logarithmic which means that as the dB increases every 10 increments, the loudness doubles. So comparing a dishwasher with a noise level of 38 to one with a level of 48 the quieter one will seem to be half as loud as the noisier one.

There may not be a good place to put a dishwasher in your kitchen. Remember the dishwasher needs to be within 36 inches of the sink. The distance requirement is there to allow good drainage into the kitchen drain pipes. A portable dishwasher may be the answer and I am not talking about your significant other that you are able to con into doing the dishes. These dishwashers have wheels and can move around the kitchen. They can add to the counter space available because of the nice 24"x24" countertop which is often butcher block so it will blend in with any existing counter material.The portable dishwasher still has to be stored. It can roll around the room and hook up to the kitchen faucet when it needs to run. The drain goes right in the kitchen sink. This is not as convenient as a built-in and it does make the sink less accessible while the dishwasher is running. However, when it gets too frustrating moving it around and hooking it up, it can finally find a permanent place under the counter top close to the sink. There are 24 inch and 18 inch versions of the portable dishwasher. Like its more permanent brother, it can also be Energy Star Certified.

Disposals

Something closely linked to the wet areas of the kitchen is a garbage disposal. Some people love them and others don't want anything to do with them. I have found them very helpful if they are used properly.

The disposal needs to be powerful enough to actually do its job. These appliances come in 1/3, ½, ¾ and 1 Horsepower (HP) versions. If a lot of your kitchen waste goes down the drain, the larger horsepower version may be in order. The stronger horsepower will also be needed if you are throwing bones down the drain.

On the other end, the 1/3 HP may well be adequate it you compost your vegetable waste and don't throw bones down the drain. If the drain goes to a septic field instead of the city sewer, a disposal is often not installed as most kitchen organic material should not be going down the drain in this situation. However I still like to specify a disposal unit because the small dregs that do go down the drain may be easily emulsified by the disposal which will help keep the drains open and the bits that do end up in the septic tank will be so broken down that the microbes can more easily digest the organics.

To get the best use and longest service from the disposal (no matter which one is selected) it needs to be operated correctly. Most all residential disposals are continuous feed systems. This means that the food items are feed in a little at a time while the water and disposal is running.

To actually use the disposal follow these steps:

1. Turn the water on full force.

2. Turn the disposal on while water is running.

3. Wash the food items down the drain to be ground up.

4. Let the disposal finish grinding then turn it off.

5. Let the water run longer (30 seconds to a minute) to flush the particulates out of the drain.

Following the above steps will keep you disposal and drain lines happy for years to come.

There are a number of manufacturers of disposals and you may want to read reviews on the brands before choosing a unit. Two companies that are known for their disposals are In-Sink-Erator and Waste King. Other companies such as General Electric and Kitchen Aid also produce disposals.

Trash compactor

I have not heard too much about trash compactors in quite a while. It seems like they were the new must-have appliance in the kitchen back in the 70's and now I rarely see them. But they are still around. This appliance may be chosen because the trek to take the garbage out is not a delightful diversion to the day, or maybe there is no trash service to your rural abode and compacting the daily load into smaller bundles may reduce the trips to the landfill.

These units can be built-in or portable just like the dishwasher but unlike that appliance the compactor does not need the kitchen sink: only electricity. Due to the low infrastructure requirements, a portable unit can be installed in the garage or utility room, away from the main part of the house. These appliances are usually about 15 inches wide (but I have seen 12 inch and 24 inch wide too) and like the dishwasher it comes in a variety of exterior finishes. A trash compactor costs about the same as a dishwasher. Pretty much the same companies that make dishwashers also make the trash compactors.

A compactor may produce from 2,000 to 5,000 pounds of force which can compact your trash up to 85%. With this kind of compaction, the trash may stay in the bin for a while before it fills up; therefore some type of odor control is advisable. Some compactors come with an odor management system in place.

Another feature to consider is a toe bar which will let a person open the compactor with just a click of the foot. This can be very handy when your hands are full or dirty. Also consider removable key-knob controls which can keep small children from turning on the unit. Some units also have an anti-jam sensor that will tell you if the compactor is too full.

Usually a garbage compactor will provide a compaction ratio such as 5:1 which means the compactor can fit the average volume of five 13 gallon bags into the one compacted compartment. Remember all those bags of trash are still in that small area so consider how much weight you can safely pick up and carry. It can get heavy.

Loudness when operating may or may not be a concern. As the unit is only used intermittently sound may not be as much as a concern as say the sound of a dishwasher. But remember as a rule of thumb that if the unit is a high capacity with a lower horsepower motor, the unit will be louder than a higher horsepower unit or even one of a lower capacity.

Maintenance is fairly simple as it should be no different than other appliances. The distance the compartment extends from the cabinet should be considered when purchasing as a full extension compartment will be easier to fill and the compressed bag easier to remove. Speaking of bags, keep in mind the ease of obtaining bags. Some units use proprietary bags that must be obtained from the manufacturer while others will work with easier to obtain generic compactor bags.

A garbage can will still be needed in the kitchen. Organic foods may be composted or thrown out the regular way or even run down the garbage disposal. If recycling is in the plans, a separate area for collecting those will be needed. Even with the need for another can in the kitchen, the compactor can make a big dent in the volume of trash put out to the street.

Cooking appliances

I labeled this section to encompass major appliances such as ranges, wall ovens, and cook tops. Microwaves will be considered in the next section. Let's review terminology. We can all generally agree that an oven is the box that heats up for the purpose of cooking food. Sometimes this oven is mounted in a wall cabinet, sometimes it sits on top of a counter as in a toaster oven and sometimes it sits below a cooktop. A cooktop is the appliance that is mounted at countertop height and has burners that a person sets pots and pans on to cook food. The confusion comes with defining range versus stove. According to Merriam-Webster a range is “a cooking stove that has an oven and a flat top with burners or heating elements”. This is why we will sometimes call a cooktop a range top. Merriam-Webster defines a stove as “a portable or fixed apparatus that burns fuel or uses electricity to provide heat (as for cooking or heating)” For a stove, think of the old wood burning stoves that were used to heat the house but a person could also set a kettle on it to heat water. I will use the term range.

Let’s talk about ranges first. These come in more variations than refrigerators. The first variation to consider is gas versus electric. A gas range is usually powered by either natural gas or propane. If you buy a gas range it is usually set up to handle natural gas. If you are using propane, follow the manufacturers recommendation on converting the range to propane. Usually there is a jet that must be replaced or adjusted. One of the best advantages to a gas range cooktop is the ability to control the heat. Control is instantaneous and very visible that is why most professionals prefer gas cook tops. However, a gas oven tends toward hot spots but an oven with convection or even a blower fan inside can help even the temperature. The broiler (yes some people still broil) is usually in the bottom pull out drawer in a gas oven.

An electric range may have exposed coil burners or the burners may be under a glass top. For an electric oven, the broiler will be in the main compartment of the oven, freeing the bottom drawer for storage. Sometimes the manufacturer calls this bottom drawer a warming drawer and that is because the oven leaks so much heat that the bottom drawer will stay warm when the oven is used. There is no such thing as an "Energy Star" range, they all leak heat.

There is another type of range cooktop that falls under the electrical category and that is an induction range. These have a lot going for them. They use an electromagnetic field below a glass cooktop which powers the element as opposed to radiant heat. The induction heats the iron in the pan directly. This allows it to come to temperature fast and also lose less heat than more conventional methods. I am talking two to four minutes faster to boil 6 quarts of water. One of the drawbacks is that there is no cue that it is on. Manufacturers are adding special lights as a cue that it is on. But there is the advantage that the element is only hot when there is a pan on it and as soon as the pan is moved the heating stops. Another quirk is that the cookware used must be magnetic. You can test your cookware by seeing if a magnet will strongly stick to the bottom of the pan. If the magnet doesn't stick, it won't work on an induction cooktop.

Another area to consider is the style; Freestanding, Drop-in or Slide-in. Freestanding is the most common. This is the range that has the 'back splash' at the rear. This back splash usually houses the clock and control displays. The electric range will have the actual controls mounted on this back splash while the gas ranges will have the controls in front so a person is not reaching over open flames to make adjustments. These backs can stick up a lot; up to 12 inches! This can have a visual impact on any decorative tile work that may be installed behind the range. However, this is the least expensive of the three styles.

Drop-in and Slide-in ranges are often confused. Look at it this way, a drop-in range is just a range without a bottom drawer or feet. A drop-in is actually mounted on a base cabinet. See it is dropped into a base cabinet. These are not often used except to replace an existing drop-in for an older home. What is actually specified more often for a new home is a slide-in. The advantage of both of these is that there is no backsplash. This makes for a nice clean application for an island or peninsula.

The second part of the range is the oven. The fuel for the oven is usually the same as for the cooktop but dual fuel ranges are available where the cooktop is gas and the oven is electric. Convection ovens are becoming more common and will usually give the option of cooking with convection or by standard methods. A convection oven can cook foods quicker or at a lower temperature but it does take some getting used to the different way of cooking.

A feature I have found useful is a double oven, specifically those that have a smaller upper oven and larger lower oven. I found myself using the upper oven more often. The smaller oven heats up faster and cooks smaller items well. The dual oven also allows a person to cook biscuits in the upper oven at one temperature and the casserole – or turkey – in the lower oven at a different temperature.

Ranges are usually 30 inches wide, but can be found in 20, 24, 36 and 48 inches with the larger sizes being of the pro-style or commercial-style. These commercial styles are also dual fuel. Many professionals prefer a gas cooktop and an electric oven. The gas cooktop allows for finite visual control while the electric oven allows for more even baking. But remember any size out of the ordinary will cost more, especially the larger ones.

If room allows it, a separate cooktop and wall oven could be useful. The wall oven may then be placed at a height that will eliminate the need to bend over when pulling hot pots out of the oven. The cost of a separate cooktop and a separate wall oven does not add together to equal the cost of a freestanding range. Plan on paying what it would cost to buy two freestanding ranges for this setup.

Microwave

The microwave oven has been around since 1954 when the Radarange was first introduced to consumers. There was a lot of wariness around the whole idea of microwaves escaping and causing harm to people. But now years later it is considered a standard appliance in the kitchen. I remember heading out to buy a microwave (my first) in 1988 but coming home with a bread maker instead (Something brand new on the market). I rationalized that I would just marry someone who had a microwave, and I did in 1990.

Microwaves have changed a lot since the 1980's. They are cheaper (something that actually lowered in price) and there is a lot more variety. Now there are microwaves of all sizes, some large enough to cook a turkey. Most even come with turntables that allow for more even heating. Most also have an electronic touch pad and some come with a child safety lock. Other options that are often seen are convection oven capability, a grilling option, defrost and reheat at the touch of a button, racks, doors that swing to the side or down, and the ability to adjust the power levels. Many even have preset buttons for things like cooking popcorn, baking potatoes or cooking a pizza; these settings will adjust power and time automatically.

There are two basic types of microwave ovens; the countertop and the built-in models.

The countertop version has a wide range of sizes from the compact versions which have about 0.7 Cu. Ft. and use 700-watt all the way to a 2.2 Cu. Ft. that use 1600-watts. The higher the wattage the faster items will heat but also the larger the oven the more wattage is needed. Physical size can also vary considerably from 10 inches tall to over 16 inches tall. Width can be from 17.5 inches to 24 inches and the unit with the door closed can take up half the depth to almost the full depth of your 24 inch counter top. Think about how you plan on using the oven and buy the right size. I have a microwave that is too short inside for my cold pancake syrup bottle to stand up.

There are several microwaves I am labeling as built-in. One is the over-the-range microwave which will have most of the same features as the countertop version but will have an added feature of serving as the vent hood over the range top. Many of them allow for a choice of venting: to the outside or recirculating. Make sure your choice will allow for your needs. These usually come in 30 inch width to fit a standard 30 inch stove.

There is one safety concern about an over-the-oven microwave. Hot dishes and cups come out of the microwave and to prevent dumping this hot liquid on to yourself the bottom of the microwave should be mounted no higher than three inches below your shoulder. For example my shoulder is at 57 inches so my microwave should not be higher than 54 inches from the floor. Base cabinets are usually 36 above the floor (that is to the top of the countertop) so 54 – 36 = 18 inches at the maximum from countertop to the bottom of the microwave for me. This may feel too low while stirring pots on the cooktop, remember the microwave may stick out more than the wall cabinets.

Two other types of built-in versions exist. One can be mounted in a wall cabinet, or a base cabinet at whatever height is convenient for the primary user. These can get very pricy. The other type is a version of this built-in but instead of a door that swings open it has a drawer that pulls out. This can be very convenient when mounted in a base cabinet.

Venthood

Just like all the other kitchen items, this one also comes in different versions. But there is some commonality such as all have more than one fan speed, most all have a removable grease filter and most come in a 30 inch and a 36 inch version. And of course they all have the same purpose, to remove the smoke, grease, odor and moisture from the cooking space.

The most common hood is the under-the-cabinet range hood. This one mounts under the cabinets above the range and may be ducted through the wall or through the roof. Some only allow for recirculating and require a charcoal filter. A light is usually integrated with the hood. Under-the-cabinet range hoods can be found in black and white and maybe a few other colors but stainless is the most popular. Be aware that there are two different types of ducts – round and rectangular, if this is a replacement hood make sure the new hood will work with the existing duct work.

If a more decorative hood is desired, a wall-mounted range hood should be considered. This one does not allow for cabinets above the range so you lose that bit of storage but it does look nicer. It still requires a wall to mount against.

An island stove requires special treatment. The hood must be one especially made for an island cooktop. An island hood is a lot deeper than the other two because the cooking fumes do not have a wall to be trapped against. This is also the reason you will need a 36 inch wide hood instead of the 30 inch for your 30 inch range. The amount of air the blower moves is also larger. For all these reasons this type of hood will end up costing a lot more than the other two, however there are more expensive versions of the other two if you really want to spend the money. This version (like the others) will usually have lights to help you see the pots on the stove.

The fourth type of hood is not really a hood and can only be used under certain conditions. This is the downdraft version. This type will sit flush with the cooktop surface and when needed, a press of a button will cause it to rise up (usually about 7 inches) and start sucking air which will be ducted down instead of up. Just like the other version, this one also has a grease filter. This vent has to be mounted in a 30 inch or 36 inch base cabinet depending on the actual downdraft vent purchased. Due to it mounting in a base cabinet, it also is only practical for a drop in cooktop not a range. Even with this limitation it can be the right choice for an island using a drop-in range top and the idea of a huge vent hood hanging down is not desired.

Want to see some fancy appliances? Go to https://akitchenyoulove.com/ch7

Chapter 8
Electrifying The Kitchen

"The whole difference between construction and creation is exactly this: that a thing constructed can only be loved after it is constructed; but a thing created is loved before it exists."
—Charles Dickens

Levels of light

There is more to electrical than hanging a light fixture in the center of the room. Most kitchens require several levels of lighting to be adequately lit. The fixture in the center of the room is the General Lighting for the room, also called ambient lighting. This is the light that goes on when you go into the kitchen in the middle of the night for a glass of water or a snack. This is the fixture that benefits being on a dimmer switch so you don't blind your eyes when you go to the kitchen in the middle of the night. This is also the one that needs to have a switch at each main entry into the room so you do not fumble around in the dark trying to reach the light switch.

The hard working layer is the task lighting. There are usually several work areas in a kitchen and each needs to be adequately lit. Even here I like to provide two levels of light. The first level is often can or recessed lights within a foot of the fronts of the wall cabinets. This light serves two functions. One is to cast light into the wall cabinets so you can find things more easily. The other is to cast light on the work surface below. The room's general light is not adequate for this. The light's position behind you when you're standing at a cabinet means it will cast your shadow onto your work surface. The overhead task light will shine on the countertop in front of you allowing a better view of the tomato you are slicing as well as your fingers that you are preserving.

The second task light is to brighten up the dark corners under the wall cabinets. The recessed lights in the ceiling are great at shining light into the wall cabinets and down to the front half of your work space, but the wall cabinet will cast a shadow below itself. Light up this space with under cabinet mounted lights. This way you can see the cookbook that is pushed to the back so you can actually work with the food items up front.

Adding glitter

Now we talk about bringing beauty into the functional space. There are all kinds of beautiful light fixtures out there. Although I am concentrating on functionality in this book, there is no reason we can't bring up looks. This is your chance to bring some sparkle to the room: use it! Splurge a little, you will only need one or two – ok, maybe three. Hang a mini chandelier over the sink or as general lighting if your ceiling is tall enough. Use a series of beautiful pendants over a bar area.

If you are dealing with low ceilings (my current little Cape Cod has 7 foot ceilings) put in recessed can lights over the sink, bar or other specialty area and buy a fancy trim for it such as the one below.

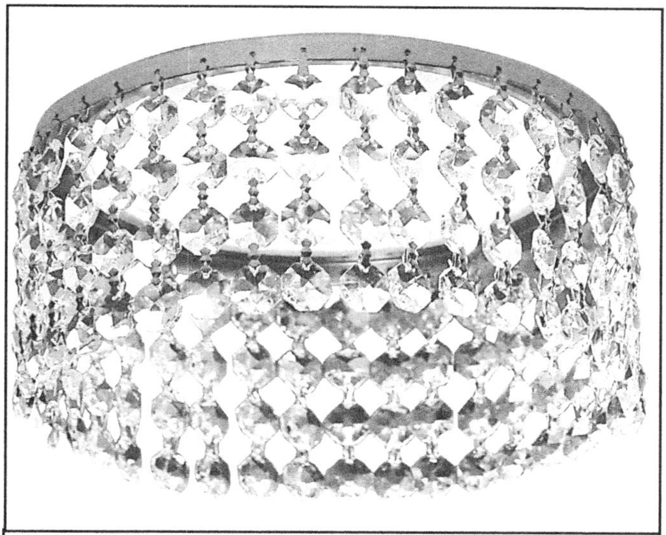

Recessed Light Trim

The above picture is from www.1800lighting.com and is their Framburg 1949 Anelique 6 inch wide recessed lighting trim.

Don't do this for all the cans because too much of a good thing loses its goodness. Just know that there are options out there. A kitchen designer can help you find them.

Controls

Each of the lighting levels above need to be controlled with their own switch: the under the cabinet lights, the recessed lights around the circumference and the general light in the center. This allows control of light level so a new layer can be added as needed. Sometimes the light from a window is all that is needed. As it gets darker more lights come on.

I like to see at least one set of lights on a dimmer, usually the general lighting or the cans. When the under cabinet lights are turned on it is because a person needs a lot of light on what they are looking at, so a dimmer on these would not likely be used. Some kitchen books suggest a dimmer on each circuit, I just think that is overkill but it can be done. But be aware that some lights won't work with a dimmer, such as fluorescent bar lights that might be used for under cabinet lights.

Another circuit that benefits from a dimmer switch is any decorative lighting, including pendants over a bar. The dimmer in this application is purely for ambiance. But lighting is a wonderful way to create a mood.

About placement, think about how the kitchen might be used. Where do you enter the kitchen? You need a switch there. If there is more than one entry into the kitchen look at putting a switch at each entry, many codes require that. On the kitchen that had four entries mentioned earlier, two entries were close together and could use the same switch but the other two entries needed switches. That is a lot of switches to install for that little kitchen. For the under cabinet lights, a single switch close to the food prep area may be all that is needed. Many people want the light over the sink on its own switch and then there are pendant island lights that will be on their own switch. The list of switched circuits keeps growing. Consider switch placement carefully. The main entry could end up looking like a sound booth control board.

Aging eyes

The eyes change as we grow older. I never have understood this aging thing. If what science says is true, that our cells replace themselves every 7 years, we should have new bodies and never get wrinkles or grey hair or dim eyes or creative hearing. But we will go on the assumption that eyes do change with time.

The extra lights on task areas: food prep, sink, stove help tremendously. So if you are thinking of cutting corners on lights and not installing those recessed fixtures or under cabinet lights; please reconsider. As our eyes age, they also start to yellow so that colors are not as sharp and bright as they once were. The extra light on items will decrease the eye strain a person may experience at such times.

Glare

This topic could easily fall under aging eyes as those are the eyes more susceptible to glare. You get glare when bright light reflects off a surface and causes discomfort in the eyes. This is often attributed to artificial lights but light from windows can be a contributor. Be sure to have a way to control window light. Curtains and blinds work well for the sink window. Shading the window from the outside naturally with trees or with a covered deck will also diffuse the light from the window. For the artificial lights inside, a dimmer switch works well. But for the under cabinet lights use a valance so the light source does not shine in the eyes while working at the counter. Any time there is potential of shining light directly into the eyes, there is potential for uncomfortable glare.

Glare can also come from a shiny counter top or back-splash. If one is shiny, choose a more matte finish for the other. Or better yet, avoid the highly polished stone or wood surfaces for these areas. Just because you are going with a painted wall back-splash, don't think you are safe. Paint comes in various sheens and unfortunately it is the higher gloss paint that is recommended for kitchens. The higher sheen is easier to clean and that is the sole purpose for it being used in the kitchen, but just be aware that the higher the sheen, the higher the reflection and so the higher the glare potential. Subduing the paint sheen with a matte counter top may be all that is needed to tone down the glare.

Bulbs

The variety of bulbs available seems to change by the day. I could spend a whole book just talking about bulbs. Let me just say that at this time there are three basic bulbs in use in the United States: Incandescent, Fluorescent, LED. There are a few other types such as Halogen but they are not used as often. In light (ha, ha) of the section on glare, LED bulbs are more prone to glare than other types.

A couple of things to know about bulbs are that they produce different color light from warm yellow to cool blue. This is known as the color temperature. What has been traditional and therefore popular in the past has been the warmer color light. That is because most incandescent bulbs produced this type of light. With the popularity of LED, any color is easily obtainable. I personally prefer the "daylight" coloring. I feel this produces a truer, less harsh color. Plants also seem to prefer this light. When that is not available I lean toward the cooler colors. The warm colors have their place in mood lighting. I have created a kitchen that combined the different lights; Fluorescent, daylight color bulbs for the general lights, Fluorescent cans lights in a warm light color and then under cabinet lights in a cooler tone. When each was turned on individually, a different mood was produced. Just remember that mixing colors so that a mixture comes on when you flip one switch, may not give the pleasing effect you want.

The second thing I want you to know about bulbs is that a change is occurring in how bulbs are rated. Incandescent bulbs were always rated in Watts which is basically the power required to operate the bulb. When Fluorescents came on the scene, they adopted the same wattage nomenclature even though they used less wattage for the same amount of light. With the popularity of LED lights, the industry is saying this 'equivalent' wattage is getting ridiculous. The LED lights require even less energy than Fluorescent so a more accurate method to compare bulbs is being used on bulb packages. The Lumen (or brightness) is now showing up on the packages.

So get used to dealing in Lumens instead of Watts when picking bulbs. The 'equivalent to ___ Watts' has not gone away but it may be on the way out.

Outlets

Residential building codes have a lot to say about outlets. However the code is fairly lax on how high to place outlets; up to 20 inches above the countertop. The optimal height of wall cabinets is 18 inches above the countertop, so this give a lot of leeway in placing receptacles where they coordinate best with the backsplash design. But the code has a lot to say about how far apart to place receptacles, what size cabinets need plugs and how many circuits there have to be. The below information applies to most codes but check your local codes before planning your outlet placement.

Outlets are usually placed no farther than 4 feet from each other on the counter top. This is to make sure an appliance is no more than 2 feet from an outlet. Counter top appliances have short cords to dissuade a person from draping the cord over the stove top or sink to be plugged in on the other side. The 4 feet spacing does not include sink and stove areas.

Any base cabinet 12 inches wide or more that is standing by itself, such as next to a sink or stove, requires an outlet. Islands and peninsulas are not exempt but do not have to follow the 4 foot rule. There only needs to be one outlet for an island or peninsula and this is usually installed on the side of the cabinet. I really feel this maybe too few for a large island so a special popup power outlet may be the answer. Just be aware that code does not allow kitchen outlets to lay horizontal on the counter, this is to prevent spills from getting in the circuit, shorting it out. Here is an example of such an outlet.

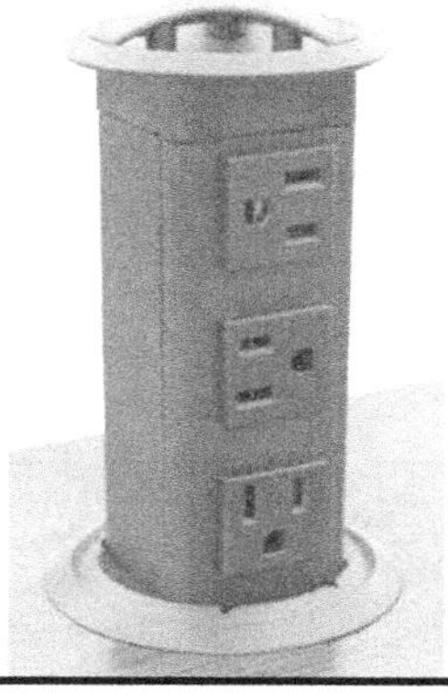

Pop-up Outlet

All outlets associated with the counter top must be on a Ground Fault Interrupt (GFI) circuit. This can be handled with a GFI Plug in the kitchen where the other plugs are wired to it in such a way that they are also protected with the GFI. Or this can be handled at the electrical panel with a special GFI breaker.

The last critical code I will mention here is that there must be two 20 amp circuits for the kitchen plugs. This can be handled in various ways. If the kitchen is being totally rewired or is a new build the plugs may be easily wired so that the top or left plug on the duplex outlet are wired together and then on the second circuit the bottom or right plugs are wired together. This way, if one circuit flips there is still one outlet on each plug that works. This is actually the preferred wiring method for many codes.

Another wiring scheme is to wire half of the kitchen on one circuit and the other half on another circuit. This way when a breaker flips, half of the kitchen is still usable.

I designed one kitchen with plug strips that have a single outlet – every 6 inches. That way there is always a plug where you need one and there are plenty of plugs. This kitchen has 44 plugs which required 3 circuits! See the picture below – the white strip above the backsplash is the outlet strip. The GFI was accomplished through GFI Circuit breakers at the electrical box.

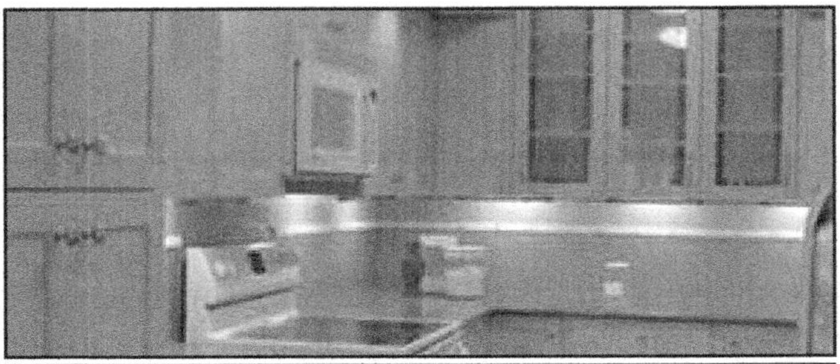

White Plug Strip Above Backsplash

Wiring for appliances

Don't forget the main electrical users in your kitchen. Each requires some sort of electrical outlet.

The refrigerator is a simple one. It can use a standard 120 volt 15-amp plug and can even be wired to one of the branch circuits feeding the plugs above the counter top. Some jurisdictions are a stickler that the refrigerator be on its own circuit but that is not in the national codes (as of yet).

The dishwasher can plug into a receptacle or be hard-wired (meaning no plug just bare wires that are wired together in an electrical box) depending on the dishwasher manufacturer. The dishwasher must be on its own circuit, it cannot be tied in with the circuits serving the countertop. However the disposal can be on the same circuit as the dishwasher. Just like the small appliance circuits serving the countertop, the dishwasher circuit needs to be on a GFI circuit.

Another appliance often over looked is the range hood. This is sometimes a plugin and sometimes hard-wired. Check the manufacturer's information. Code usually requires this to be on its own circuit.

The Oven and Cook top or Range can be the hard core users of electricity when they are electric and not gas. A standalone electric range is usually a plug in, but be careful here, there are at least two versions of plug out there for ranges. Make sure you use the correct one for your appliance and check for code compliance.

Windows and skylights

Any living space is enhanced with windows. It is recommended that most rooms have light coming from windows on adjacent walls, this lends more depth and even lighting to the room. And let's face it, most of us feel better when we can see sun light. If at all possible, plan for a window in the kitchen. If this is not possible, maybe a view of the outside is still available by opening the kitchen to another room. If all else fails there are skylights and light tunnels. I really discourage people from cutting holes in their roof. The more holes in the roof, the more chance there is for a leaky roof.

Although I advocate windows, remember what I said about glare above. Just be aware and plan for light control through that window to reduce glare.

The Electrician is your friend

If this is too much for you, call an electrician. Call sooner rather than later. Where I live, the trades are so booked up it may be 3 months before one can work on your project.

Electricians are very knowledgeable about the local codes and may even be able to suggest things that will keep your cost down. If nothing else, invite an electrician to lunch or dinner and pick their brain about your project. Just be sure to pick up the tab.

To see the pictures in this chapter in color and other inovative lighting ideas go to https://akitchenyoulove.com/ch8

Chapter 9
Behind The Walls

"Great ideas need landing gear as well as wings."
—C. D. Jackson

History

Plumbing inside the house is actually a fairly recent phenomenon when compared to the whole history of mankind. I understand Rome had a pipe system with running water in the 3rd century AD which supplied over a million people with water. Other areas in the Roman Empire were so captivated by Rome's success that they created their own aqueduct systems. These systems were so reliable and durable that a few are still partly in use.

Talking about more modern times, my Uncle John did not have plumbing in his house and he passed away in 1988. I understand that when his mother was alive, there was a tank set up outside the kitchen that collected rain water off of the roof and a single tap was installed in the kitchen so she did have running water of sorts until the tank broke down.

The water I remember from my uncle's place was from a well (really a cistern) in the front yard. This well collected rain water off the roof, I guess it just replaced the tank outside the kitchen. My mother would not drink the water because she said she had fished too many cats out of the cistern (I never asked her if they were alive or not). I thought it was the best water I had ever tasted.

The cities did receive plumbing much sooner than the country and my Uncle lived in the country. The cities had to deal with the masses and sanitation and illness due to lack of sanitation so they were forced into acting and setting up a system of bringing water in, and sewage out, of the city.

But when did hot water start being common? According to Wikipedia, the first gas water heater was invented around 1889 by Edwin Ruud, a Norwegian mechanical engineer who had immigrated to Pittsburgh Pennsylvania. In fact the Ruud Manufacturing Company is still in existence today making tank-type and tankless water heaters.

There are two main parts to a plumbing system; the supply and the drain.

Supply

The supply brings water into your house from the city main or from your own well system. In the house it usually heads straight to your water heater where it splits off, some goes into the water heater and the rest (or cold side) goes to all the various cold water taps in the house.

In the recent past the supply lines were made from galvanized iron pipes. This was popular up to the 1960s. The original pipes from the city main into my current house were galvanized. This house was built in 1957; when we purchased it in 2015 we replaced the plumbing, because the corrosion scaling was so bad that the only water tap that flowed was the hot water side in the downstairs bath tub!

After the 1960s, copper became the pipe of choice for water supply lines. The copper was much more malleable than the galvanized pipes, meaning it could bend and so was easier to install through walls in one run with no joints. The 'no joints' was important as each joint is a potential leak waiting to happen. Copper has its drawbacks too, the main one is that it can kink when being bent and that will restrict the flow, think of a water hose with a kink. Copper has also become very, very expensive as of this writing. But don't worry, a new material has appeared.

PEX is a relatively new product: PEX stands for polyethylene crosslinked. Very bendable, it can be snaked through most walls and small areas without kinking which make it a very versatile water line. This tubing can be obtained in three basic colors; red, white and blue. Often the incoming supply line will use the white PEX, the red is reserved for the hot water line and blue for the cold. This is an easy product to work with and the fittings are easy to attach with a minimum investment in tools. Even a do-it-yourselfer could re-plumb a house with this system.

Drain

All this water has to go somewhere and that somewhere is down the drain. Draining away the unwanted water has come a long way from pouring it out on the ground. Now it is moved to sewage treatment plant whether that is in a big city or in a septic tank in your own yard. Just like with the water lines, the modern plumbing has progressed through different materials. Cast Iron was the material of choice for a long time. However the houses from the 1960s and 70s are starting to see corrosion eating through the pipes. Sewage is actually a corrosive. I had a plumber that was pumping my septic tank tell me he had seen concrete lids on tanks eaten away from the corrosive nature of the sewage fumes.

The little Cape Cod we bought and totally re-plumbed had a drain made from something called Orangeburg. We had never heard of it but it was popular during the post war housing boom because other drainage materials were scarce. Considering that Orangeburg is like papier-mâché made with asphalt, it has held up very well. When we uncovered it, the pipe was no longer round but rather oblong so we replaced it.

At this time the most common material is PVC pipes. This serves well but is a stiff non-bending material. Drains have one requirement that you must know about if you are going to mess with them. A straight run of drain must have a slope of at least ¼ inch for each foot of run but no more than 3 inches per foot. Less than ¼ inch will cause headaches with constant clogged drains but more than 3 inches will cause the liquid water part of the sewage to run ahead of the solids and the solids will not have a chance of washing down with the liquids. Of course that does not apply for vertical pipes.

Venting - the hidden pipe

This is the one pipe that can cause the most trouble in a remodel. You may have access to the water supply lines and the drain pipes from a crawl space or basement but the vent pipe runs through the walls and exits out the roof. Often other vent pipes from other plumbing fixtures are attached to a single vent pipe in the attic in order to cut down on roof penetrations. So if a remodel calls for moving the kitchen sink, a whole new can of worms is opened up.

The vent pipe cannot be easily moved. The purpose of this pipe is to regulate the air pressure in the waste pipe system so the water will flow as it should. All fixtures like sinks, tubs, showers, and toilets have a p-trap. Look under the kitchen sink and you will see a bit of pipe that looks like a "P" lying on its face. The purpose of this curved pipe is to hold water (so always have something to catch the water when removing this pipe). This water acts as a plug for sewer gasses coming the other way. The vent provides an air break which allows the water to stay in the trap. If the vent is clogged or if there is no vent, all the water will flush down the system, not sticking around, and then sewer gases will enter the house. Or the water will not be able to flow into the drain pipe, causing it to back up or drain very slowly.

The Vent has to penetrate the roof for almost the same reason. Sewer gasses will exit the top of the vent pipe and we do not want that gas exiting into the attic or the wall.

Island sink

As mentioned earlier all fixtures that drain water must have a vent and that vent must be within so many feet of the fixture as specified in the code. Kitchen sinks are usually mounted in a cabinet against a wall, often with a window above it. The vent pipe can usually work around the window. But what about a sink mounted in an island or peninsula?

There are special ways to deal with this situation. The first choice is to use an Air Admittance valve (AAV). These are a one-way valve which opens when water is being discharged down the drain; this allows air to enter the system to allow pressure to equalize in the pipe. The valve then closes when the pressure is equalized and sewer gasses cannot get out. This valve is mounted under the sink past the trap and as high as the area will allow. These nifty little valves can really save the day – or sink, but not all jurisdictions will allow them.

If the AAV is not allowed in your area another alternative does exist. An Island Fixture Vent, sometimes called a "Chicago Loop" is a possibility. The following picture explains the system.

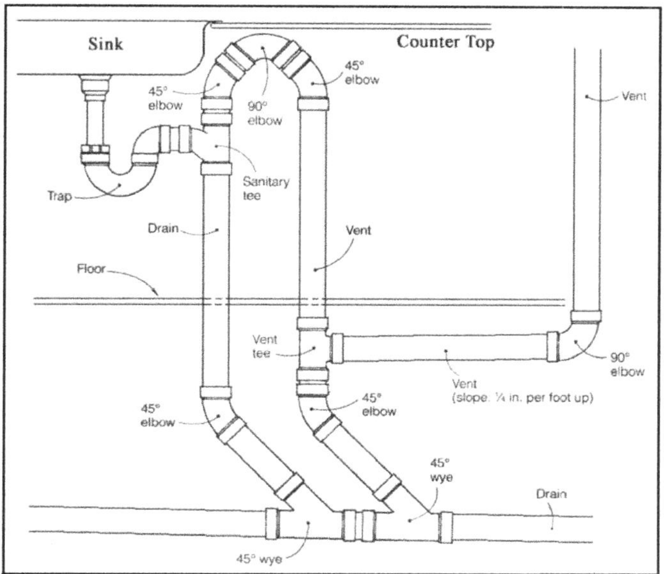

Chicago Loop

Image credit: Wikipedia.com

This type of venting does require more piping and a lot more labor to install that is why the AAV is preferred.

I just wanted you to know there are work arounds for most situations but they often require more time and money – the AAV being an exception.

Water softeners and purifiers

Hard water seems to permeate the United States. What makes the water hard is the naturally occurring minerals in the water, calcium and magnesium being the main culprits. Rain water is naturally soft and does not contain such minerals, it is when the water seeps into the ground through all those layers of rock that the water collects the mineral. The more minerals present, the harder the water. A water softener will remove most of these minerals.

Hard water can be a problem as the minerals will precipitate out and cause problems for water fixtures, build up deposits in pipes, clog water heaters (a big one), cause undue wear in valves such as washing machine fill valves, and leave unsightly deposits in sinks.

The ion-exchange resin devices are the most widely used device to remove the minerals for household use. This works by exchanging the calcium and magnesium ions for sodium ions hence the name. The resin must be re-charged using a sodium chloride or sodium hydroxide solution.

Some people are concerned about the salt introduced to the water through a water softener. Those on a sodium restricted diet may consider a reverse osmosis system for drinking and cooking water. Other people don't like the way soap seems to cling to the skin and feels difficult to rinse off with soft water.

Take heart if you do not want to go with a water softening system, there are some benefits to hard water. Hard water reduces the solubility of potentially toxic metal ions like lead and copper which end up being more soluble in soft water.

A water softener removes calcium and replaces it with sodium whereas a water purification system does much more. These terms are not the same. Water purification usually uses a reverse osmosis, distillation or deionization system. A high quality filter system will remove the calcium like a water softener but also many other chemical contaminants such as chlorine, arsenic, pesticides and various other troublemakers.

A water purification system can be a whole house system or just a point of use such as at the kitchen sink.

The choice is yours. If the main problem is scale and soap scum then a water softener may be your best choice. If your water taste or smells funny you may want to consider a water purification system. If you are on a public water system, they will be able to provide you with a copy of their latest water analysis. Look at that and then decide what you want to do about your water.

Your friendly plumber

Just like with the electrician, your plumber can be your best asset. A good plumber is knowledgeable about the local codes and may have tips and advise on how to deal with problem areas. Seek them out before starting a project involving plumbing. Ask friends for referrals of plumbers who know their trade. Just like with electricians, a good one will be booked out several weeks or even months so get in there early.

For additional information check out https://akitchenyoulove.com/ch9

Chapter 10
Tying It Together

"When love and skill work together, expect a masterpiece."
—John Ruskin

Form follows function

Now you are ready to really start planning. Start by sketching your ideas on paper or use a software program.

First measure all the walls, if there is a doorway or a window, measure to the frame. What you want is the usable wall space available for cabinets. Draw the walls to scale on the paper. A good scale is ½ inch equals 1 foot. If using standard paper, tape sheets together or use large pieces of paper.

Start drawing in your cabinets. Remember cabinets come in 3 inch increments and don't forget you can use spacers. If the physical floor space where your new kitchen is to go is clear (no cabinets currently there) draw the outline on the floor with chalk or use painters tape. Then play in your kitchen. Does the spacing feel right for you? Are all the critical areas only a few spaces away? Pretend you are working in the kitchen, preparing a meal.

Now comes pretty

Most people think of the looks of the kitchen before the actual layout. You may already know how you want it to look; the cabinet's color and materials maybe even the brand, the countertop material and color and also the backsplash. As shown previously, there is a lot to consider.

For ideas, look through websites such as pinterest and houzz. Save pictures that appeal to you. What exactly is it that you like about each. More than likely everything you like will not fit together in the same kitchen. Remember that the more elaborate the look, the more expensive it will be.

Style of home

The style of your home will play a big part in what the kitchen will look like. Some typical styles include: Traditional, Cape Cod, Craftsman, Farmhouse, Mediterranean, Midcentury, Beach, Contemporary, Asian, Rustic, Ranch, Scandinavian, Southwestern, and Victorian. There are many others that I will not list but you get the idea. If the home being remodeled does not have a distinct style now may be your chance to give it some style. If one of the above appeals to you investigate it further.

Each of the styles above will have its own ambiance. However one cabinet door style may work well in several of the home styles. For example the single flat panel cabinet door has very clean lines so it works well with Contemporary, Eclectic, Modern, Asian, Industrial, Midcentury and Scandinavian. What may set it apart in each style are the color of the doors and cabinets and the hardware used. That is where the separation from Midcentury and Asian occurs.

If your home is Victorian but you are really taken with the clean lines of a Midcentury there is a conflict. My inclination is go with what you really want but keep in mind when you try to sell the house the potential buyer will see the Victorian on the outside and will expect Victorian on the inside. So the decision is yours.

Working with a designer

The above confusion can be straightened out when working with a designer. A designer can see potential problems and develop solutions. At the initial meeting the kitchen is discussed extensively and all the measurements are taken.

One thing I do with a new client is to hand them homework. I want to know how they use their kitchen, what they expect to store in the space and what they consider to be 'must haves.' Some of the worksheets may seem rather personal, asking about height and weight and mobility issues. This information is needed to create a space that fits their specific needs. Someone who has problems bending will benefit from drawers and roll out shelves so they do not have to bend down to find things.

Some of the worksheets tell me where the owner expects to use an item and how often it is used. A blender is a good example. Some people will use a blender close to the sink for easy cleaning. Others may want it close to the refrigerator so smoothie ingredients are at hand. Someone else may only use it occasionally and want it stored away.

A designer takes all this information and uses it to develop a plan. A preliminary plan or two will be presented to you - the client. This is sometimes called the concept phase and the drawings the conceptual drawings. When one design is settled on, including changes, the conceptual drawings are completed and presented to the client. These are great for a dream board or when construction is still months away. The perspective views make it easy for you to visualize the space.

The next step would be to create dimensioned drawings and specifications. These include fully dimensioned drawings and elevations, mechanical plans, construction plans if required, electrical plans and final perspective drawings. Your contractor will require these to create the finished space. Specifications are also included but will be very general unless the material selection packet has been agreed upon.

Working with a contractor

After the plans are accepted, a contractor or installer is engaged. If the project is large, requiring many trades such as electricians, plumbers and carpenters a project manager or general contractor may be required. If it is just a matter of removing old and installing new cabinets, countertops and backsplash an installer may be the way to go.

The designer – myself – can hand the project off to your contractor after the design work has been accomplished. I also offer services overseeing the project. Working in this capacity, I can ensure the plan is followed and I will be available to handle any unforeseen problems that may arise. If all that is needed is installation, I can find an installer for you.

What can you do yourself

If money is an issue, there is much that can be done to keep the cost down. Consider doing some of the work yourself. Often the demolition can be handled by the owner or the owner and a hired handyman, but don't do the home-show thing and demolish with a sledgehammer! It is safer and easier to finesse the cabinets down, usually intact where they can be reused or donated. Also the cabinets can be installed by the owner if they have experience with do-it-yourself projects. Both the base and wall cabinets have to be shimmed and leveled and screwed into the wall framing. The screws must attach to the framing! If you are not comfortable with doing this, hire an installer. Sometimes you can act as a helper on the job for a reduced rate. The countertop should be installed by a professional because it requires a high degree of specialized skill and special tools.

After the base and wall cabinets are installed, call in the countertop salesman. The countertop is such a critical piece to get right and the countertop retailer knows it is so they usually include the cost of installation in the cost of the material. The base cabinets have to be installed before they measure for the countertops. The countertop installers usually install the sink but leave connecting the plumbing to someone else.

After installation of the countertop, the backsplash can be installed. This is another area you may choose to handle yourself. If you are not confident, practice on a scrap piece of drywall first.

Parting words

This is not rocket science, and any mistakes you may make can be patched, repaired or repurchased. Have fun with the process. Don't stress out. Enjoy eating out for several weeks (or months). Remember the TV shows where they do this in 3 days are just that, a show. A good job that will last and work properly takes time.

Enjoy your new kitchen. If you need help contact me through my website annskandb.com

To see some sample forms I request new clients fill out go to htps://akitchenyoulove/ch10

ABOUT THE AUTHOR

Kitchen and bath designer Ann McKinley was born in Newport News Virginia and grew up in Friendswood Texas, a small suburb south of Houston. Her passion for housing started at a young age while living in one of the first houses built in a new and growing neighborhood. Wandering through the houses as they were being built sparked a desire to create beautiful and functional living spaces. Since growing up, Ann has always been involved in housing in various ways. Her passion has taken the form of owning rental properties, volunteering with Habitat for Humanity, building an airport community, designing and building her own home, rehabbing worn out houses and working as a Texas Realtor. And now her passion shines with designing kitchens and bathrooms. Ann is uniquely positioned with a degree in Mechanical Engineering and experience with remodeling which she uses to her and her clients advantage in understanding the mechanics of a house and knowing what goes on behind the walls. Ann currently lives in Gordonsville Virginia with her husband and assorted cats.

You can learn more at:

Website: AnnsKandB.com

Facebook: fb.com/annskandb

Made in the USA
Monee, IL
04 November 2026

67384897R00098